Terminal Ca
People with

Ruth Sims RGN, DNCert, Dip NAMH
Chief Executive

Veronica A Moss MBBS, DTM&H,
DCH, DObst RCOG
Medical Director

Mildmay Mission Hospital
London

Edward Arnold
A division of Hodder & Stoughton
LONDON   MELBOURNE   AUCKLAND

Dedication

To all those people with AIDS whom we have come to know and love, and especially to those who have lived with us at Mildmay.

© 1991 Veronica Moss and Ruth Sims

First published in Great Britain 1991
Second impression 1992

British Library Cataloguing in Publication Data

Sims, Ruth
 Terminal care for people with AIDS.
 1. AIDS patients. Care
 I. Title II. Moss, Veronica

 ISBN 0–340–52877–X

Whilst the advice and information in this book is believed to be true and accurate at the date of going to press, neither the author nor the publisher can accept any legal responsibility or liability for any errors or omissions that may be made. In particular (but without limiting the generality of the preceding disclaimer) every effort has been made to check drug dosages; however, it is still possible that errors have been missed. Furthermore, dosage schedules are constantly being revised and new side effects recognised. For these reasons the reader is strongly urged to consult the drug companies' printed instructions before administering any of the drugs recommended in this book.

All names of patients in this book have been changed to protect their identity.

Typeset by Butler & Tanner Ltd, Frome and London
Printed and bound in Great Britain for Edward Arnold
a division of Hodder and Stoughton Limited,
Mill Road, Dunton Green, Sevenoaks, Kent TN13 2YA
by Biddles Limited, Guildford and King's Lynn

Contents

Foreword

The global pandemic of AIDS and HIV Infection continues to escalate in all countries in which this disease has been reported. The WHO estimate (in 1992) that by the year 2000, up to 10 million people will have AIDS, and up to 40 million people will have been infected with HIV. In the United Kingdom 5,782 AIDS diagnoses had been reported by the end of March 1992 and 17,494 had been confirmed HIV-1 positive.

AIDS is today the greatest threat to the public health in our life-time and has presented us with unique challenges. For the caring professions, these challenges have most frequently focused on the need to offer competent, confident and compassionate care for those thousands of often frightened individuals requiring medical and nursing support. To do this effectively, health care professionals need an opportunity to extend their skills and knowledge, and space to explore their own attitudes to the highly charged issues which AIDS demands we confront. One of the most difficult issues requiring exploration is our response to death and dying.

Death is part of life and dying is simply 'living the end of life'. My own experience in caring for people with AIDS has reminded me of the common wish we all have to 'live the end of our life' well. To support patients with AIDS 'living the end of their life' well requires skill and an awareness of the unique needs of individuals nearing that end. These include the need to be safe and not to be hurt, to be given refuge or sanctuary, and to be comforted and the need to be accepted, to belong and to give and receive love.

This important book is about meeting those needs. It is not about death but about 'living the end of our life' well. It describes a unique model of care which has been created by Ruth Sims, Veronica Moss and their colleagues at a rather special hospital in the East End of London. The on-going dynamic experiences of the Mildmay Mission Hospital are charting a path through our fears and confusion in relation to offering quality care to individuals seeking support for an appropriate end to their life.

It describes a sensitive and comprehensive approach to the practical issues involved in meeting the terminal care needs of individuals with AIDS. Like its authors, this book reflects love and hope and provides for the first time the expert guidance needed to be with our patients in a meaningful way as they confront the final stage of their lives.

We are all going to have the experience, many times over before this epidemic has run its course, of knowing and loving individuals 'living the end of their life' with AIDS. This book shows us how to do it and I commend it to all health care professionals.

Robert J. Pratt RN, BA, MSc, RGN, RNT, DipN(Lond).
Vice Principal/Head of Faculty
Faculty of Continuing Education
Riverside College of Nursing, London
1990

AIDS reports to WHO at 1 April 1992
(NB. represents serious underreporting)

Africa	144,863
Americas	268,445
Asia	1,442
Europe	65,875
Oceania	3,523
Total	484,148

Introduction

Why a book on terminal care for people with AIDS?

Much has been written in recent years both on terminal care in general and on AIDS in particular. The general principles of terminal care, as practised in traditional hospices and through such home support services as those provided by Macmillan nurses, are well established. Knowledge about AIDS and of how it takes its inexorable toll on human lives, is growing day by day. So is there a need for a book which deals with terminal care and AIDS?

We believe that there is such a need. The advent of AIDS has challenged science to find answers very quickly. It has also challenged health care professionals to examine firmly held beliefs about, and attitudes to, all patients or people in their care as nothing else has done this century. AIDS is also challenging us to re-examine many of our attitudes to terminal care. And since as yet there is no cure, the emphasis must be on care – at home, in hospices, and in hospitals.

Another reason for writing this book is the conviction that, sadly, in the next few years the number of people affected by AIDS will continue to grow. It will become increasingly necessary for primary care teams in the community to take on board the continuing and terminal care needs of people with AIDS in the community. The time will soon be here when most General Practitioners will have at least one or two people with AIDS on their books, most district nurses will have someone with AIDS requiring nursing care at home, and most people will know someone who has been touched by AIDS through bereavement. As has already happened in America and in many parts of the Third World, increasing numbers of women and children, whole families and communities will be affected.

When compared with deaths caused by other modern 'epidemics', such as road traffic accidents, heart disease and cervical cancer, the number of deaths resulting from AIDS is still relatively small. However, when the rapid spread to date and the frightening prevalence rates that are now being reported in the USA and in many parts of the Third World are considered it is clear that there is no room for complacency.

This is particularly true when considering young heterosexual people who have, in the main, not accepted the need for changes in the attitudes to casual sex that have been part of Western culture since the 1960s. It is even more true when thinking about those who are addicted to drugs who often take double risks – sexually and through the sharing of needles.

There is also a need to dispel some of the fears and prejudices that are still so evident among some health care professionals. Many others are prepared and willing to get involved, but are apprehensive of the unknown. There are many similarities in the terminal care required for people with cancer and that required for those with AIDS. However there are also major differences (see Table i) which we hope to clarify.

Table i Common features of AIDS which are likely to differ from those of the terminally ill patient with cancer.

1.	Predominantly younger age group.
2.	Multi-systems disease which may result in
	— blindness
	— paralysis
	— neuropathy
	— confusion
	— myopathy
	— skin disorders
	— severe diarrhoea.
3.	Misery of many co-existing physical problems.
4.	Large number of drugs being taken.
5.	It is often difficult to identify the terminal phase of the disease – very sick patients may improve and opt for acute treatments.
6.	Treatments such as blood transfusions, total parental nutrition, and IV therapies are often given to maintain quality of life in terminal care.
7.	Lengthy dying process – patients may be unconscious for a week or more.
8.	Most people with AIDS know more about their disease and its treatment than the people caring for them and demand involvement in their care and treatment.
9.	Fear, prejudice and lack of compassion are evident in many parts of society.
10.	Social isolation of patients and their families.
11.	Homelessness or inadequate housing.
12.	Need for long-term supervisory care and housing for disabled people.

Our aims

In writing this book we aim to increase the awareness of health care professionals to the issues surrounding terminal care for people with AIDS. We hope this will enable them to make more appropriate responses to the needs of those who come to them for help. We hope, too, that the practical guidelines given will enable them to make those responses with confidence. The practical guidelines and general principles are based on the experience we have gained during the past five years. Since January 1987 we have been responsible for researching, planning, and establishing Europe's first AIDS hospice and continuing care unit at Mildmay in the East End of London. This includes day and home care provided by a multiprofessional team. We have learnt most from those who are living with AIDS – many of whom have been our patients. We have also learnt much from their families, friends and partners. We have witnessed tremendous courage and devotion, and have felt the challenge to re-examine our practice and attitudes in relation to all client groups. We pass this challenge on to you.

Acknowledgements

Many people have helped and encouraged us in the writing of this book and we would like them to know how much their encouragement has been appreciated.

In particular Robert Pratt, Vice Principal, The Riverside College of Nursing of London, without whose encouragement and advice this book would probably never have been written, and Mrs Taylor-Thompson, the Chairman of the Mildmay Board of Directors, who, from the very beginning, has been entirely enthusiastic and supportive in our venture.

A number of colleagues have encouraged us or given advice related to their particular speciality: Barbara Dicks, In-patient Services Manager, Royal Marsden Hospital and a member of the Board of Governors of Mildmay; Shirley Lunn, Hospice Counsellor, Ann Wood, Clinical Nurse Specialist, and Peter Clarke, Chaplain, all at Mildmay; John Atkinson in Glasgow; Dr Ray Brettle and Dr Jacqueline Mok in Edinburgh; Dr Diana Gibb and Candy Duggan at the Hospital for Sick Children, Great Ormond Street; Dr Colin Murray-Parkes; David Miller; Peter Harwood, Senior House Officer at Mildmay; Richard Wells, Head of Rehabilitation, Royal Marsden Hospital and AIDS Adviser to the World Health Organisation; our many friends in Frontliners, in particular Peter Tillson and Kevin Rimmington from whom we have learnt so much. We have also learnt a great deal from Body Positive and Positively Women.

We would like to thank all the staff at Mildmay for their support, especially our Personal Assistants, Dorothy Hannan and Shirley Jones, for their very practical support and hard work in preparing the manuscript. We are grateful to them for their patience in dealing with corrections and alterations while continuing to perform their duties with their usual efficiency.

Notes to readers

Gender   The person with AIDS may be a man, woman or child, but for ease of reference the words he or him rather than the more cumbersome he/she or him/her has been used throughout this book.

Family   Included in the term 'family' is anyone who is important to the patient – a partner, anyone related by blood or marriage, or a close friend. By partner we mean the person to whom the patient has the deepest commitment; the one who is acknowledged as the present partner is the one nominated by the patient as such. It may therefore refer to a husband, a wife, a common law husband or wife, or a lover.

Counsellor   This word is used to refer to anyone who has a training in counselling and who has formal commitments to the work of counselling. This may refer to a social worker with counselling remit, a psychologist as well as to the person who has a recognised training in counselling.

*What this book is **not** about*   This book is *not*
— a text book on AIDS
— a text book on how to be a counsellor, how to nurse etc.
— a book about education or prevention of AIDS

This book does not pretend to have all the answers. It does not try to deal with any subjects that are outside our experience. It is a book which simply seeks to share the experience and understanding gained during the past five years from talking with, working with, and living with people with AIDS. Much time has also been spent talking with and learning from other health care professionals involved in the care of people with AIDS. Many of the experiences are of our own personal experience; but none of it has been in isolation from the rest of the team. For all in the multiprofessional team at Mildmay it has been a time of learning together. Of course there is still much to be learnt.

This book does not enter into issues related to politics or debates about lifestyles   We do not believe that the terminal care arena is appropriate for such debate. Suffice it to say that we believe that no person should be discriminated against in any way; all are deserving of the highest standards of care, given with genuine love and acceptance, and backed by sufficient funding and manpower to enable each person living with AIDS to do so with dignity and in the place of his choice.

'*Patients*'   Our consumer research indicated that people with AIDS in our care setting were comfortable with the term 'patient'. They were familiar with it as recipients of care in hospitals or the community and saw no reason to be called anything else.

Abbreviations

Abbreviations used in this book (see in particular Chapter 6)

Dosages and administration of drugs

bd	twice daily; alternatively bid
BM	bowel movement
4 hourly	to be taken every 4 hours; alt. q4h
h	hour(s)
IM	intramuscular
IV	intravenous
Kg	kilogram
l	litre
lb	pound
mg	milligram(s)
ml	millilitre(s)
mm	millimeter(s)
mmol	millimole (s)
min	minute(s)
μg	microgram(s)
NSAID	non-steroidal anti-inflammatory drug(s)
nocte	at night
PO	per os; by mouth
PR	per rectum
prn	pro re nata, 'as required'
qds	four times in 24 hours; alt. qid
s–c	sub cutaneous
sl	sub lingual
stat	at once
tds	three times in 24 hours; alt. tid

1 Where to care

In the United Kingdom the options available for the terminal care of people with AIDS falls into two main categories:
— *hospital care* and
— *non hospital care* which, for the purpose of this text will be classified as *community care*, i.e.
  home care
  sheltered accommodation
  hospice care.

Care in the hospital

At the present time the majority of people with AIDS who need care choose to be cared for by staff at designated AIDS centres in major cities. The reasons for this are many but include:
— the belief that the very best in care is provided only at these centres;
— there they will be accepted and need not fear the rejection and prejudice associated with their diagnosis and
— they can preserve their anonymity in a way which they could not do if using local services.
Despite the increase in numbers of people with AIDS this is still the case, especially in London. Beds in designated AIDS wards are full, and often as many patients as are in the ward are disseminated throughout the same hospital into general wards, under the care of the consultant in HIV disease. This would account for the fact that many health care professionals working outside of major cities may never have met or cared for a person with AIDS, indeed they will have seen nothing of the reality of the growing demand for services.

A recent survey has shown that the majority of people with AIDS still die in hospital (Kennedy, 1990). For many patients, especially those who have had repeated hospital admissions, this is entirely appropriate. The security of being cared for in familiar surroundings by people who may have known the patient since he was first diagnosed, and who clearly care for and about the patient, cannot be underestimated. For some people the maintenance of hope that comes of being in an acute care setting is essential if living, for them, is to have quality. For others the availability of emergency treatment, if needed, helps to allay fears.

Care in the community

Bill was 32 years of age. He was a person with AIDS living in San Francisco – and he was dying. At over six feet tall he was painfully thin, weighing only a few stones. He looked like an old man, emaciated and balding.

I first met Bill in a small dark room in what I can only describe as a broken down hotel. The curtains were pinned together at the window and Bill was wearing dark glasses. Everything was dark and dismal. A kitten was jumping around the room, as were fleas, and there were cockroaches on the table and in cupboards. Bill was huddled in his bed looking wretched.

I saw many patients in similar surroundings in San Francisco. Would they not have been much happier in the airy light and comfortable surroundings of the Coming Home residential hospice?

For them, I was told, it would not have been better. The thing Bill valued most was his independence, the ability to control his own life and surroundings, to make decisions and to retain his dignity. His experience was that this was in no way possible to any similar extent in any care providing institution.

In spite of living in squalor community care was right for Bill.

Martin was 24 years of age. He was a person with AIDS – he was dying.

He had occupied an acute bed in a London hospital for several weeks and the decision was made that he should be discharged to his parents' home where they would care for him. Martin had not lived with them for seven years. They could not handle the fact that he was gay, especially as they did not want him, as they put it, influencing his two younger brothers and turning them 'that way'. He had lived for the past four years with his partner John, who had cared for him in the flat they shared prior to Martin's admission to hospital. John had not been allowed any input into the decision made regarding Martin's discharge and Martin was too weak to fight his parents.

When Martin went to the family home he was emaciated, incontinent of urine and faeces, had oral and oesophageal candida and was thoroughly wretched and depressed. He was very withdrawn and spoke very little.

The statutory and voluntary services were called in with input from the General Practitioner, District Nursing Services, Social Services (home help) and Crossroads Care Attendant Scheme. His nursing care was excellent, his symptom control good and voluntary help enabled his parents to cope. His parents, however, were concerned that his two younger brothers be protected both from Martin and his lifestyle. John was never allowed to visit their home.

Martin died after ten days, without the love and support of the person who mattered most in the world to him.

For Martin, although input from statutory and voluntary services was good, some of his most fundamental needs were not met and community care was not best for him.

What is community care?

Is it being at home with family who care about you and are prepared to give that caring practical expression, asking for very little outside help?

Is it home care given mainly by professionals and volunteers with input from friends and family?

Or is it similar to the following experience.

A young man lives alone in his London flat refusing all care save the help of his buddy. AIDS has been scored in the wood of his front door — it is sad to see the desperate, unsuccessful attempts he has made to obliterate it. He refuses to go out for fear he will be attacked. He is not receiving care from statutory services; he is afraid of who might be sent to care for him.

He has experienced so much rejection and persecution that he just cannot risk it again.

Sadly, there are people, including health care professionals, who would justify these very fears.

In providing appropriate terminal care it is essential to identify needs: needs as perceived by the patient and those important to him. Provision and choice of care should therefore be in response to those needs. In order to identify needs it is essential to involve patients, giving them relevant information and choices. It should be remembered that many people in the terminal stages of the disease will be suffering from dementia; whenever possible in the planning of care, options should be presented to the patient and those important to him, and liaisons established as early as possible.

The Government White Paper 'Caring for people' describes Community Care in the following way:

Community care means providing the right level of intervention and support to enable people to achieve maximum independence and control over their own lives. For this aim to become a reality, the development of a wide range of services provided in a variety of settings is essential.

Care at home

Care at home involves caring for the patient and those important to him as a unit. When it is successful, care provided in the familiar surroundings of the home, with multi-professional input from the statutory and voluntary services, can produce the very best of terminal care. In the freedom of their own homes independence is often more easily maintained and people can behave as they wish. When home care is the appropriate option it should be available and accessible to everyone who needs it.

Care in sheltered accommodation

For people who are increasingly facing homelessness and are chronically ill but still self caring and not requiring nursing care, there is a great need for sheltered accommodation. At the present time this need remains unfulfilled in England except for a very few initiatives. Provision is being planned in some areas by voluntary organisations, private individuals and by housing associations. A number of these are also seeking to provide homes for people in the form of flats or rooms within houses.

In this situation supervision is often necessary, with a 'warden' or person on call, as is the provision of one hot meal per day. Special accommodation need not be necessary. The clients have similar needs to any chronically sick person, but the diagnosis of AIDS may result in rejection from general provision.

The provision of sheltered accommodation for people with AIDS is an identified gap in service provision, especially in areas such as London where there are large numbers of people with AIDS who require care.

Care in a hospice

For some patients, hospice care will be the most appropriate, whether it be in a traditional hospice or a designated unit such as the Mildmay or London Lighthouse. The circumstances include when:
—   the patient is living alone
—   there is poor symptom control
—   there are frightening symptoms.
Hospices will need to be able to offer 24 hour multiprofessional care. *Time* for patients, time to care, time to listen or just time to 'be there'; this can only be achieved with high staffing ratios.

The advantages of hospice care include:
—   living in a homely setting
—   the privacy of a private room but the opportunity to share communal facilities
—   continuing care including respite, rehabiliative and convalescent

care, referral back to acute centres and support and counselling
for partners and families
— bereavement support and follow up.

Day care facilities

The aims of providing a non acute day care facility as part of the
continuum of care are:
— to enable people to remain at home for as long as possible; and
— to enhance the quality of life of patients and their carers.
To achieve this the care on offer should include:
— treatment facilities
    palliative and maintenance only
    assistance with bathing and personal care
    emotional support and counselling
    dental treatment
    chiropody
    rehabilitation including physiotherapy, occupational and art
    therapies, etc.
— provision of hot meals
— welfare advice and help
— respite for patient and/or carer
— recreational facilities
    films, concerts, visiting artistes
    crafts
    hairdressing.
'Traditional' hospices offering day care may make their facilities available to people with AIDS.

Having looked at the options for care and what they offer, what are
the possible problems relating to these options?

Problems with hospital care

Understaffing and the high dependency of patients in the acute hospital
may make it difficult for carers to have time to look after people in the
way that they would like. Input to the families, partners and friends of
the patient in terms of support, help and counselling is usually limited.
Bereavement support and counselling is often non-existent. Many
patients with AIDS are in need of terminal care for weeks or even
months with resultant pressures on staff and on the demand for beds.

Problems with community care

Problems with home care

Can 24 hour care be provided when it is needed? In the United Kingdom it has seldom been possible to provide 24 hour care patients other than for those suffering from advanced malignant disease, and then demand for services has far exceeded supply. Can spans of care for 4–8 hours be provided to enable the primary carer to go out to work? Are district nurses trained and ready to give the intravenous (IV) drugs and total parenteral nutrition becoming more and more necessary in palliative care for people with AIDS? Who will give the tremendous input of skilled counselling needed by these patients and those they love? Can bereavement support and follow up be provided to families at home?

Problems with care in sheltered accommodation

At present people living in sheltered accommodation are not always linking up with local statutory and voluntary services, resulting in problems when residents become acutely ill or when those with chronic illness need skilled nursing rather than supervisory care. Planners of care need to ensure that, at the very least, there is an informed and sympathetic General Practitioner who is willing to take the residents on to his or her list. It is encouraging that in some areas of London planners of hostels and half way houses are involved in joint planning committees, liaising with and developing local services.

Problems with hospice care

For some patients hospice care may be unacceptable. For some it signifies the end of the line: 'No more can be done, everyone has given up on me'. This option must be presented with considerable sensitivity. Hospices offering respite and convalescent care help to allay fears that people admitted to a hospice are there to die.

Many traditional hospices, that is those caring mainly for patients with cancer, are either unable or unwilling to admit people with AIDS. The reasons for non-acceptance include:
— funding is/has been given only for patients with cancer
— inadequate facilities; unable to cope with demand for beds from people with cancer
— management level decision
— hospice staff unwilling or feel unqualified to care for people with AIDS.

Whatever the reason given, the outcome is that there are patients travelling miles from home to receive care that could much more appropriately be given nearer their home.

Wherever the care is offered the *aim* should be the same – *to give care that is responsive to the total needs of the patient and his family, i.e. physical, emotional, spiritual and social needs.* All carers share the same concerns. With hospitals and hospital wards closing the pressure on acute beds is increasing. This results in earlier discharge of patients into the community without proportionate transfer of funding and resources. This, together with the earlier discharge of post-operative patients, patients from acute elderly rehabilitation wards, and the emphasis on community care for the disabled, is increasing the demand for all community services. The current overstretching and underfunding of community services, with the inevitable low morale leading to understaffing, could result in diluted services and have a devastating effect on the quality and range of community care.

Many areas are tackling the problem, setting up educational programmes and support for staff, liaising, appointing advisors and/or specialist teams, researching need and investigating new initiatives. There remains, however, much to be done if we are to be able to offer options, real choices, for care to the projected numbers of people with AIDS who will die in this country this century.

Mark's story

Mark was in his early twenties. He came with his mother to 'have a look round' before deciding whether he wanted to be admitted to Mildmay. He was referred for 'terminal care'. Mark had ideally wanted to stay at home but that was not possible as his mother and father worked and he was too frightened to spend long periods of time alone. He decided he would come to Mildmay and was admitted the next day. He was suffering from peripheral neuropathy and atypical Mycobacterial disease.

Within 24 hours of admission Mark developed a severe abdominal pain and the team felt that he should be offered the opportunity of returning to his acute centre for investigations and possible surgery. Having been made comfortable, Mark was seen by the doctor and his primary nurse who discussed with him the options and likely outcomes. He asked if he could have two hours to decide and requested that the local Roman Catholic parish priest (a man not known to him) visit him. He talked with the priest and was given the last rites. At 4 pm Mark told the team that he had decided that he wished to have no further acute interventions. He knew that he may die quite soon but that was his choice and he told his parents of his decision. Over a period of 24 hours it seemed that this young boy had become a man.

Mark did not die; in fact, he lived for a year – his condition stabilised and, for a time, he improved a great deal. This time was very important to him and his parents, a time during which they, with the help of the counsellor and the whole multiprofessional team, worked through painful issues and emerged with an openness and honesty that they as a family had never known before.

Mark never lost sight of his wish to die at home and his mother felt guilty that she was out at work and felt unable to care for Mark at home. However, Mark decided he would like to go home for the odd day at the weekend. This was arranged with attention to detail so that the whole family felt supported and had adequate back up. Then Mark developed Cytomegalo virus (CMV) retinitis – he had dreaded this possibility because, apart from the deteriorating vision, he was needle phobic.

Mark again looked at his options and decided he could not risk going blind, and would therefore opt for having intravenous Gancyclovir infusions. He returned to his acute centre to have the Hickman line sited. By now his mother was more confident about his visits home, his relationship with his father was much better and Mark really wanted to spend weekends at home. But the infusion … his parents felt quite unable to take it on, he would have to go home just for odd days. Community care of his intravenous infusion was not available. Mark took control of the situation – he still wanted to die at home but his condition was deteriorating and he knew this. Needle phobic or not, Mark decided that he would learn to give his Gancyclovir and flush his line. He felt that he needed the freedom to control his environment rather than, as he saw it, having the environment control him. His mother was also taught to give the infusion and gradually they both became more confident. She had decided by now to give up her job so that she could care for Mark at home. The home care nurses visited Mark and his family on the unit and he was glad to establish relationships. His discharge was carefully planned so that he had several trial weekends before finally going home. He regularly contacted the unit to let the team know how he was. His mother cared for him with only the minimum of input from community services. This was as Mark wanted it. After 12 weeks at home Mark died peacefully. His parents were well supported by the home care team and the priest who was now their friend.

Mark did take control of his life. He made choices with outcomes that his family and the staff found difficult and challenging, and overcame tremendous personal fears and obstacles to make his wish to die at home become a reality.

References

Government White Paper (1989). *Caring for People – Community care in the next decade and beyond.* CM 849. HMSO, London.

Kennedy, A. (1990). Communicable Disease Surveillance Centre, Public Health Laboratories. (Unpublished).

2 Responding to the terminal care needs of people with AIDS

People with AIDS have a need to *live* with AIDS, and not just to sit, or lie, around waiting to die. The Oxford English Dictionary describes 'to live' as meaning 'to be alive'. This living can embrace a broad spectrum from, at the one end, a meaningless miserable existence to, at the other end, living with quality.

The Wilkes (1980) report states:

'The main aims of those providing terminal care should be to improve the quality of daily life by removing or alleviating unpleasant symptoms and helping to prevent the patient from suffering fear or loneliness.'

'Quality' means different things to different people. Some people enjoy eating whole foods, others enjoy pie and chips. Some people find talking helpful, others find it difficult. People are individuals, all with differing needs; the response to those needs must therefore always be individually tailored.

Who is this person with AIDS whose needs the carer is attempting to address? It is the man, woman, teenager, child or baby who has been referred to the hospital, hospice and/or community services and needs care. The person with AIDS is someone with a multi-systems disease who, in common with all individuals, has needs which must be met if health is to be maintained, needs that must be responded to if that person is to be able to live.

Quality of life can only be maintained and improved if distressing symptoms can be relieved and, recognising the potential that each individual has, working with or for them to maximise this potential. Assumptions about what constitutes quality for individuals should not be made – for some people at certain times quality will mean being allowed to choose to opt out.

Physical needs

As AIDS is a multi-systems disease, its presentation in terminal care is varied and often complex. The patient in the advanced stages of the disease may be ulcerated from mouth to anus causing difficulty in eating and swallowing. He may be emaciated, having torrential diarrhoea of several litres a day. He will be weak and tired and may look prematurely old, displaying purple skin lesions over many parts of his body.

The physical care of these patients presents great challenges to carers, not least the need for good clinical management. The problems commonly encountered are:

— total body pain
— neuropathy
— myopathy
— weight loss, often as much as one-third of body weight
— dyspnoea
— nausea and/or vomiting
— diarrhoea
— skin lesions
— severe debility and decreased mobility
— intermittent confusion and inability to maintain personal safety.

Responding to physical needs

AIDS commonly affects people at a time in their life when they would have been at their most creative and productive.

It is essential to work *with* the patient and important that, whenever possible, control is where it belongs – with the patient. Prior to admission many patients will have been cared for by their partner or a family member. It is essential that the partner and/or family member is encouraged to continue to be a key member of the caring team if they and the patient wish it, and provided they are not needing respite themselves.

In order to give control to the patient it is necessary to give information relating to options available. This places considerable responsibility on carers in an area of care which is constantly changing and developing. Having encouraged the patient to make choices it is essential that his wishes are respected. This can be difficult for some carers who may usually be directive in their approach.

It could be argued that for too long care professionals have not listened to their patients; care professionals *alone* have been the assessors, and the care given based on their assessment.

> A friend of mine, who is a doctor, was admitted to hospital for major surgery. Less than 24 hours post operatively he asked for an injection as he had severe pain. He was told, 'It can't be that bad yet, you only had an injection 2 hours ago.'

Pain, nausea and discomfort should be as the patient feels it, not as the doctor or nurse thinks it is or should be.

Patients need comfort, that is the physical freedom from discomfort.

The response of a multiprofessional team of carers is the best way to achieve this.

Highly skilled medical care must be provided, with input from the doctor as necessary, often on a daily basis. To maintain symptom control (see Chapter 6) it may be necessary to resort to polypharmacy in order to control the many distressing symptoms the patient may have. It may be difficult for doctors in general practice to keep up this level of care for more than one or two terminally ill people at a time, especially over long periods of time. Good symptom control is dependent on effective communication between doctors and nurses (see also Chapter 3).

Highly skilled nursing care with attention to detail is essential. Sometimes the nurse's role is to encourage, sometimes to 'push' a little, but always to be there when needed. Patients need to maintain their independence and skill is required to offer help without pressurising and to give choices, space and time to the patient. Some patients may refuse care and in these cases their wishes must be respected; this may be difficult for the nurse to accept and will often have implications for carers, partners, family and friends. Nurses must know about the disease, its treatment and issues relating to research. Many of the patients will know more about the disease than those caring for them and they will need to discuss issues with their carers. The nurses' skill, knowledge, attitudes and standards of care must give them credibility with their patients (see also Chapter 4).

Input from *rehabilitative therapies* is likely to be invaluable in terms of restoring and maintaining physical function.

At times it may be necessary to give treatments not normally given in a terminal care setting, for example the use of

— Intravenous Gancyclovir (daily five days per week is the usual regime) to prevent progression to blindness in patients with Cytomegalo virus (CMV) retinitis

— Total Parenteral Nutrition (TPN) to selected patients with Cryptosporidial diarrhoea and to some with obstructive Kaposis sarcoma

— Nebulised Pentamidine as a prophylaxis against *Pneumocystis carinii* pneumonia once every two weeks.

The above are maintenance therapies initiated in acute centres and, in some areas, the treatments are maintained in the community. When the human immunodeficiency virus affects the brain, the resultant dementia will render increasing numbers of people unable to maintain their own safety and independence. Even in the ideal situation it is impossible to provide literal 24 hour care – the minute you turn your back the patient will fall! There will always be an element of risk which has to be accepted, as the cost to the patient of total safety would surely be unacceptable.

Emotional needs

The emotional environment is created by people interacting with the patient, people demonstrating that they care and showing unconditional love and acceptance (see also Chapter 7). The needs for love, acceptance and security are particularly important in this care setting as many people with AIDS will have experienced rejection for much of their lives. This rejection may have caused them to leave the family home, physically separating themselves from all people, family and 'friends', familiar to them. Loneliness and isolation can be difficult and destructive and, in desperation, people often make disastrous choices, perhaps leading to unfulfilling relationships and apparent promiscuity. Carers should beware of imposing feelings of inappropriate guilt on the patient.

With the diagnosis of AIDS people may experience many losses:
— loss of control
— loss of dignity
— loss of body image
— loss of a future

and an anticipated loss of any and everything that is important to them. Rejection, isolation and guilt may compound the feeling that the person is useless, hence their self esteem is lost.

Fears may be expressed, fear of dying, of the process and of what happens after death. Coming to terms with death and dying is painful even for those who have lived a full life but it must be so much more difficult for the many young people with AIDS.

The need to maintain hope

Absence of hope equals hopelessness and this is something that care professionals and their patients should not accept. There is never 'nothing that can be done'.

> A friend had a biopsy of a lump in her breast. The result took ten days to come through. During that time she had gone through the various scenarios in her mind from the worst to the best. She felt she worked through a lot of issues but was very strong about this. 'The one thing I could not tolerate was them saying there is nothing they could do; I could not survive without hope.'

The need for honesty

In any caring situation mutual trust is essential and patients need to know that those caring for them will not mislead them or be dishonest with them. The degree of openness and discussion relating to sensitive issues is dependent on knowing the patient and respecting his wishes.

The choice as to what information is disclosed, and the things that are better left unsaid, should be guided by a knowledge of the patient's coping mechanism.

The need to raise difficult and painful issues

When the patient trusts his carer it will be easier for the patient to raise difficult and painful issues. However, it is essential to recognise that some people's coping mechanism is found in denial (see Chapter 7). The patient may well be aware of their situation with all its implications but the last thing they want is to talk about it.

> A young man who was experiencing short term memory loss would often ask members of the care team, 'Do I have AIDS?' He would move from reality to denial and finally back to reality. In the end he said, 'Did you know I have AIDS? Isn't it terrible, I hate it.'

He needed honesty coupled with re-assurance that his worst fear of dying alone would not become a reality.

The need to overcome feelings of isolation

As mentioned at the beginning of this section, patients need freedom from isolation, rejection, guilt and fear. The isolation felt by people with AIDS is probably something that few others have experienced to the same degree.

> Peter, a patient with AIDS said, 'As a person with AIDS I feel isolated when I am with well people'.

> A female patient said that when she was told of her HIV status, the most pressing need for her was to meet other women who were HIV Ab positive. Despite being surrounded by caring staff she felt alone in her pain and misery.

Not only do patients need reassurance that they will die comfortably and with dignity, with their wishes respected through dying and death, but also that they will not be alone.

The need for encouragement and motivation

In providing encouragement and motivation to help the person with AIDS get on with the business of living the personality of the carer is of great importance. There are patients who will do anything for a particular nurse and other nurses will just not achieve the same results. The carer must be flexible in his or her approach and remember that it is what the patient wants and needs that matters.

The need to be valued and to be of value

Every person cared for is of value and contributes much that is of great significance. The following was stated by Maria Swafford, a nurse working with AIDS programme in San Francisco:

'We enter the lives of our patients at a very special but traumatic time — when they are confronting their imminent mortality. Often bonds of profound intimacy are forged through these trying circumstances and in the midst of tragedy care givers can facilitate opportunities for incredible emotional and spiritual growth by their patients and their families.'

The need for the carer's time

Time spent performing tasks, listening or just time to be there are all important. Even when patients appear to be unconscious perhaps by just being there and holding a hand they can be reassured that they are not alone and given a sense of being cared for and about.

In order to respond to patients emotional needs carers, whether statutory or voluntary, must have the following skills.
— The ability to listen and respond and also to know when to be silent.
— The ability to be able to find out where the patient 'is' regarding his situation i.e. what he has been told and what he feels about it. It is important not to respond blindly to questions but rather build on what is known and work with the patient at his pace and in his time.
— The ability to recognise when it is necessary to refer to someone with greater skill; for example do not adopt the role of a trained and experienced counsellor unless qualified to do so.
— Carers must ensure that confidentiality is maintained; sharing something that has been told in confidence must only be done with the patient's permission.
— The ability to be able to love and accept people as they are. Attitudes toward people shows in non-verbal communication long before any word is spoken. Sincerity and a genuine desire to care will be recognised; insincerity may be difficult to tolerate.

> A young man with AIDS asked why so many people who met him for the first time felt it necessary to hug and kiss him. 'Is it this touch thing gone mad?' he said.

> A young girl patient said that she had terrible stomach ache. 'If you stopped stuffing yourself full of cream toffees and pepsi cola you might feel better,' I replied. She stared at me for a minute, then laughed and said, 'Yeah'. We were always straight with each other and it made the relationship real.

As with all relationships it is not necessary for carers to agree with all aspects of the patient's life to love and accept them. Responding to patient's emotional needs and helping them to deal with unfinished business will often be the release they needed and give them the freedom to get on with living.

Social needs

In responding to the social needs of people with AIDS it is important to liaise with social workers involved with the patient to identify the history and the current situation. Patients may have been involved with a social worker for some time and it is vital that, whenever possible, these links are maintained.

Housing and accommodation

The lack of suitable housing is a very big problem for the person with AIDS who:
— is homeless; they may have been homeless prior to becoming ill or have been evicted or asked to leave their accommodation for a variety of reasons including their diagnosis, their lifestyle, their colour, inability to pay rent, or in arrears with mortgage payments
— is unable to live alone
— lives alone but needs help
— can no longer climb flights of stairs and needs ground floor accommodation
— has become terminally ill and decides to sell his property or move from rented accommodation but then recovers
— for the sick mother and her baby in bed-sit accommodation.
It is often difficult to find accommodation for homeless people and there is no quick and easy way to solve this problem. Homeless people with a diagnosis of AIDS should be dealt with immediately wherever they are.

When caring for people with AIDS it is important to find out what the situation is regarding housing in their area and having done so to establish personal links with key personnel. In some areas housing associations are coming forward and expressing a willingness to house people with AIDS, either within general provision or in designated units. In Edinburgh the statutory services are selecting, training, and funding families who take people with AIDS into their homes. Training programmes for home helps can provide carers who are confident, and assistance that is both flexible and appropriate.

Hospitals with patients with AIDS should be flexible and allow well babies and toddlers to stay with their sick mothers. Assistance may be bought in from agencies for nursery nurses to be available for the period of the stay. Those involved in planning care should give thought to enabling families to stay together when the parents need care.

There are several organisations that may be able to give small grants to patients to assist with housing. These include the AIDS Care Education Trust (ACET), the Terrence Higgins Trust, Frontliners, Mainliners, and Body Positive. (See Appendix 1.)

In major cities the cost of accommodation for families and friends who may wish to visit a patient can be prohibitive. It is desirable for centres caring for people with AIDS to offer the opportunity for family or friends to stay overnight in the patient's room and/or to provide accommodation (e.g. an apartment or room) within the centre.

24-hour care

Is home care really an option for those people with AIDS who are living alone and need 24-hour nursing care or 24-hour supervisory care?

For those living alone and housebound a considerable amount of assistance with shopping, cleaning and food preparation may be needed from home helps and/or volunteers. A mother with AIDS may need help in caring for her baby – at the moment this help is usually given by friends.

Finance

People with AIDS need to know the allowances that may be available to them and how to gain access to these allowances. Benefits from Social Services and grants from charitable agencies may be available, and include:
— Housing Benefit
— Mobility Allowance
— Attendance Allowance
— Social fund – crisis loans
— Sickness Benefit
— Income Support
— Invalidity Benefit (after 28 weeks)

Further information may be sought from the Department of Social Services, ACET and THT. See also Appendixes 1 and 2.

Many patients may also have fears and anxieties for the future of their partner and family, especially if they have been the main provider of income or they are a single parent. Carers should be able to reassure the patient and to advise on the benefits and income support systems available.

It is important to recognise when a patient may need financial help, not only to provide for their own (and their families') everyday needs such as food and accommodation, but to help in maintaining their quality of life. For example, most people with AIDS will have lost a considerable amount of weight and be demoralised by having to appear in ill-fitting clothes which emphasise the altered body image – the ability to be able to purchase new clothes may have a very positive effect on their morale. Patients may also gain pleasure from being able to afford to buy a small present for their carer(s) or a member of their family.

People with AIDS may be sharing mortgages or rents with their partner or family member and may need advice and assistance in sorting out the legal and financial issues involved.

Spiritual needs

When people are ill and activity is restricted they will often, for the first time in many busy years, have time to reflect about the meaning and purpose of their life. This may be a painful process and involve them in examining areas of guilt and conflict as well as contemplating their value and belief systems. Many will need help and support from their carers during this time (see also Chapter 8). Given a safe, secure, loving environment free from pressure, ridicule and judgemental attitudes, people will feel more able to explore and express their spiritual needs, conflicts and problems. People's religious beliefs, or the fact that they have no religious belief, must be respected.

Carers must recognise that

— Patients need to have the freedom to worship according to their faith and this should be facilitated whenever possible

— some patients will need to have the sacraments brought to them, others will derive great comfort by being taken to a place of worship

— the need for pastoral care may be met by the Hospital Chaplain or by another spiritual advisor of the patient's own choosing

— the patient may need to discuss issues relating to his funeral service.

Patients must not be pressurised regarding their spiritual needs, but it is important not to neglect this area of care. Patients may experience a need for forgiveness of themselves, of others, and a sense of being forgiven by God and/or others before they can find peace of mind.

Until people with AIDS know that they can trust the carer, and that acceptance of them and friendship to them is genuine, the carer will not be in a position to share with them issues relating to their most fundamental needs.

Reference

Wilkes, E., Harnett, G., Speed, D. *et al.* (1980). *Report of the working group on terminal care*. HMSO, London.

3 The multiprofessional team

'So in everything, do to others what you would have them do to you'
Matthew 7:12

When the declared aims of care are to provide for the needs of the whole person it is not always possible, or even good, for one person to provide all the care. One person does not usually have the expertise or the time that is needed. It would also encourage too great a dependence on one person; when that particular carer is unavailable or fails in some way, it is possible that the whole care package can fall apart. At their best, multiprofessional teams can ensure that all the needs of the patient are met. The team must have a common approach and understanding of the overall aim, but team members must also have an understanding of, and respect for, each other's expertise. Good communication regarding each profession's codes of conduct and policies, as well as about subjects directly related to the care of a particular person, enables the team to work together with mutual respect and understanding. This can be achieved through regular multiprofessional team meetings, at case conferences where appropriate, as well as through the use of the telephone or in direct discussion with the appropriate team member.

Aims of care

Each individual team member will have their own philosophy or belief systems which will affect how the care is delivered. However, to achieve a coordinated approach it is important that the team as a whole agree on the overall aims of care. The aims should include the following.
— To provide for the needs of the whole person.
— To treat each person as an individual, with respect and acceptance, acknowledging each person's right to privacy and confidentiality.
— To give control back to the patient as far as is possible.
— To enhance the quality of life by good care, including aids for daily living, appropriate housing and effective symptom control, enabling the patient to live life as fully as possible until death.
— To facilitate a comfortable and dignified death.
— To provide support and bereavement follow up to families, partners and friends, recognising all who are of importance to the patient.

The multiprofessional team

Ideally, the core of the team should include nurses, a doctor, therapists, a dietitian, social workers, counsellors and psychologists, and chaplains and ministers of religion, either to give regular in-put or to be available when needed or wanted.

Nurses

The nurses, together with the partner or family of the patient, provide the greatest in-put to care of the terminally ill person with AIDS. Professor Eric Wilkes in his report on the working party on terminal care in 1980 commented, rightly, that good terminal care depends, in the main, on good nursing (Wilkes, 1980). Nurses are privileged to provide the most intimate details of care, and are also the first to whom the patients will turn for advice or for a listening ear. Nurses are also in a good position to observe and monitor symptoms and developing problems, as well as the response to symptom control management and medication. In the community in Britain, the district nursing services have for many years worked with the primary nursing model, ideally with the primary nurse as the coordinator of the care given to any one patient. Good communication between the nurses and doctors is of the greatest importance in order to achieve good symptom control and medical management. Nursing issues are dealt with in Chapter 4.

Doctors

The doctor's role and medical issues are dealt with in more detail in Chapters 5 and 6, but suffice it to say here that the doctor is but one member of the team and should communicate closely with other members of the team, in particular with the nurses. The doctor's most obvious roles here are in symptom control and the management of medical problems directly related to AIDS. However, the doctor should also be available to the team for advice and discussion in order to contribute to the whole, as well as being available to each individual patient and his family to give information, advice, and support. When the patient dies the doctor has practical matters to deal with, such as death certificates and cremation forms, but he should also be available for on-going support to the family who may have questions and worries that need to be dealt with.

Therapists

Physiotherapists have an important role to play in maintaining quality of life for as long as possible, in easing or comforting distressing muscle aches and pains, and in relieving some of the breathing difficulties related to chest infections. They may also have a great deal to contribute to such problems as seating, lifting, and those related to the chronic disabilities that often occur with the slowly progressive neurological forms of the disease. Some patients who appear to be moribund may recover and then require rehabilitation with very active physiotherapy in-put.

Occupational therapists also have an important role, and, in liaison with physiotherapists, may help to achieve a great improvement in the quality of life through improving functions and activities of daily living, enabling the patient to maintain independence for as long as possible.

In-put from therapists can be invaluable in the community, enabling the patient to live at home through the use of adaptations or aids that are available for daily living. Other therapies should also be available according to the needs and wishes of the individual patient; for example art therapy may not only provide stimulation to creativity, and occupation, but may also enable the patient to express feelings and emotions that he is unable to talk about.

Dietitian

Dietetic advice is, of course, an important aspect of the overall care for the person with AIDS. As the illness progresses eating difficulties may increase. Some patients may experiment with a variety of diets, hoping to combat the disease and its progress. Some diets undoubtedly contribute to the development of malnutrition, particularly in those who already have persistent and severe diarrhoea, as occurs in cryptosporidiosis. As the illness progresses and becomes more debilitating problems of nausea, dysphagia or intractable vomiting may develop and total parenteral nutrition (TPN) may be instituted. It is quite possible to maintain TPN in the community, but good liaison is essential between the dietitian, the doctors, the pharmacists and the laboratory involved. In these cases difficult decisions as to how long TPN should be continued in the terminal care setting will need to be faced (see also Chapters 5 and 6).

Social Workers

Many of the social needs of patients with AIDS have been discussed in Chapter 2. As the illness progresses, and as patients become more debilitated or disabled by neurological problems such as caused by HIV encephalopathy, cerebral toxoplasmosis and progressive multifocal levcoencephalopathy (PML) (see Chapter 6), housing, financial and general support and supervision needs may become more and more difficult to deal with. Single parents who have small children may worry about their children being taken into care, or about what will happen to their children when they die. Financial problems may be weighing very heavily and will require sensitive handling. The complexities of welfare benefit, legal problems, funeral expenses and the making of wills may all seem very daunting; sorting these out may make a very big difference to the quality of those last few weeks or months of life. Psychiatric social workers may be involved together with psychiatrists in sorting out problems that have arisen as a result of developing HIV encephalopathy, such as the disinhibited, sometimes manic behaviours that may be an early sign of dementia even in the late stages of the syndrome. In some hospitals and hospices, and sometimes in the community, social workers may be involved in counselling, in liaison with psychologists and psychiatrists. There may be serious family conflict over wills in which the social workers or counsellors may find themselves having to take on the role of mediators (see also Chapters 2 and 7).

Counsellors and Psychologists

Strong counselling in-put will be needed, both to the patient and to those close to him, to provide support during the patient's illness and also bereavement follow-up and counselling as necessary after death. Counsellors and welfare assistants need to work very closely together, as some of the counselling in-put deals with the matters discussed in the above section on social work. However many issues relate to death and dying, to family conflicts, and to relationships which are often very complex, such as an ex-spouse and children visiting a patient whose present partner is also visiting and between whom there might be considerable antagonism. Parents, particularly fathers, have often not been able to accept their son's gay partnership. (Many of these issues are looked at in more detail in Chapter 7.) The work of the counsellor or psychologist will often overlap into spiritual or pastoral care as patients express deep conflict, doubts, anger, guilt and fear. It is important that counsellors and psychologists recognise the contributions that the chaplain or ministers of religion have to make in this area, and that each respects the other and works together with the patient to achieve peace of mind.

Chaplains and Ministers of Religion

Spiritual and pastoral care issues are dealt with in Chapter 8. These should be seen as having an important contribution to make to the whole care of the person who is living with AIDS, particularly as he enters the terminal phases. This is the time when the person needs strong reassurance, understanding, empathy, simple friendship and access to those important sacraments or rituals that reinforce a sense of belonging and of confidence. Uncomplicated and unconditional acceptance and love, creating a sense of security and of trust between the patient and his spiritual adviser, will enable the patient to explore doubts, fears, beliefs or non beliefs without fear of ridicule or rejection. However, the barriers will remain firmly up if he senses condemnation, judgement or even fear of the illness itself on the part of the chaplain.

A team which communicates and is well coordinated has the potential for providing very high standards of care. However, with such a number of people involved the potential for confusion is also great. The patient may not be able to, or wish to, relate to so many people and may prefer to communicate deeply with only one or two members of the team, or may find his support elsewhere. Someone who has recently become blind, or who is severely debilitated and ill, may become totally confused and withdrawn if he is being forced to relate to too many people. In this situation it is important that the team agrees amongst itself who is the best person to be the key worker. This is likely to be the primary nurse but it could be anyone with whom the patient communicates well. It is important also that issues of confidentiality are understood and respected within the team. The patient may not be at all happy about matters that he has discussed with one person being passed on to the rest of the team. Anyone who has been the recipient of sensitive or confidential information should always check with the patient first before divulging the details to other team members.

Categories of care

The continuum of care in advanced disease is non acute and different categories of care may be required. These categories include:
— respite care
— rehabilitative or convalescent care
— terminal care
— bereavement support and follow up (this is most commonly offered in the home or in a hospice).

Respite care

For patients being cared for at home, particularly those who are severely debilitated or disabled, respite care may provide a much needed and sometimes essential change, not only for the patient but also for the carer. For the patient respite care may provide an opportunity for time and space on their own, but with all the necessities of life being cared for by a professional team in the comfort of a hospice or nursing home. For the carers it may provide a break from the exhaustion of continually caring for someone close to them. Regular respite admissions every six to eight weeks may enable someone to remain at home through most of their illness, particularly if this is taking a slowly progressive form. Respite may also be provided on a day basis once or twice a week at a day centre. In admitting patients for respite care it may become apparent that the patient is terminally ill and in need of more intensive nursing care and support than that which is possible to provide in the community. Admission may then need to be arranged in response to a crisis situation.

Convalescent and rehabilitative care

Patients requiring convalescence or rehabilitation will be recovering from an acute illness or an apparent terminal phase (patients referred for terminal care may recover and require rehabilitative care). Physiotherapy and occupational therapy in-put is particularly important in this group of patients. Physiotherapy may also be of value in the day care or home setting for patients who have had neurological problems.

All these categories of care provision will be increasingly necessary during the next five years, even in the unlikely event of a cure or vaccine being found within the next few years. Patients requiring long term care or continuing care – people who are seriously debilitated or disabled by the virus, people who may have permanent neurological problems such as HIV related encephalopathy, hemiplegias or severe neuropathy – will present particular problems in the community.

Sheltered or supervised accommodation, or accommodation adapted for disabled people is already desperately needed, especially in the larger cities. Continuing in-put will be required from all health care professionals, with intensification of in-put from time to time, particularly as people become terminally ill.

Patient directed care and the multiprofessional team

Good team work may result in excellent provision of care. However, it must always be remembered that the patient is the hub of the wheel and should, as far as possible, be in control at all times. There is also, as has been mentioned, the potential for confusion, manipulation and misunderstanding particularly if communication breaks down between team members and the patient, or the patient plays one team member off against the other.

A patient in our care appeared to be very confused, and also had all of us confused. We eventually found out that there had been more than 20 people or agencies involved in his care in the community, most of whom did not know of the others existence until a meeting was set up to which the patient was also invited. The patient appeared to be in control, but was in fact suffering from the early effects of HIV encephalopathy.

Patient directed care in practice and at its best means that the patient is in control, working with the different members of the multiprofessional team who inform, advise and enable him to make valid choices out of the available options. The options available will vary from time to time and the patient's ability to make choices will also vary according to his health, both physical and emotional. Many professionals, particularly doctors and perhaps nurses, are used to being directive in their approach to patients. At times the patient prefers or needs directive care and skill is required to know when this is appropriate. Sometimes the patient makes it clear that this is what he wants and then his wish should, of course, be respected, unless the patient is abdicating all responsibility, thereby increasing his dependency and illness.

A patient admitted for rehabilitation was very demotivated and unwilling to cooperate with any attempts at rehabilitation. At first his need to be left alone and to abdicate responsibility was accepted and respected; however, it became clear that this attitude was seriously affecting his progress and health – he was not terminally ill. He was challenged from time to time by different members of the team to take up that responsibility again for himself. A consistent approach had to be developed by the team and he was eventually able to take up the responsibility, take part in the case conference and discharge planning, and eventually to go home.

In practice, patient directed care means that ward routine has to be flexible, sometimes with a considerable amount of negotiation between patient, nurse and other patients to ensure harmonious communal living. It may mean that times for visits from physiotherapists or counsellors may have to be negotiated with the patient to fit in with other plans that he may have. It means that the patient is given whatever information he needs or wants in order to be able to make informed choices. This includes information regarding medication – some patients know a great deal about the different medications that they are taking, particularly those related to AIDS, for example Zidovudine. Patients with AIDS will often be very informed about the latest research into new drugs, for example drugs that are available in America but not in the UK, and herbal or other remedies which are being tried in various countries. Doctors and nurses in particular need to keep themselves well informed in order to be able to discuss the pros and cons of a particular medication or regime.

Inherent in this approach to care is a risk that the advice given may be rejected, the care or even the carer may not be wanted or appreciated. This can be particularly difficult for care givers to accept or understand. Professional carers are used to patients being grateful, passive and cooperative. Patients who are not, are quickly labelled difficult, or sometimes even psychotic.

A patient who refused a number of investigations and treatments that were being advised and who had been travelling to and from hospital frequently and felt himself to be deteriorating, refused to accept any further active intervention. He felt that he was being pressurised, by the doctors, against his will, became very angry when he was referred to a psychiatrist and walked out. His partner was told that he had become psychotic and needed psychiatric intervention and possibly admission to a psychiatric unit. His partner eventually found him wandering around the streets of London in a very exhausted state, brought him home and persuaded him to come to Mildmay for some respite on the understanding that he would not be forced into anything that he did not wish to have done. For the first few days he was extremely suspicious, very withdrawn and refused all nursing and medical care including any medication. If asked if he wanted a drink or food he would say no. He was in total body pain and had severe oral thrush, which made his mouth sore and swallowing difficult. The doctor, on introducing herself was asked why she thought she knew what was best for him and was told to get out. Nurses were told that they were not wanted, he only wanted to be left alone. It was clear that he was very angry and suspicious, and he needed time and space to himself in order to build up some trust in what we had to offer. The nurses and the doctor continued to go in from time to time to explain briefly that he did not need to continue in pain and that his mouth could be made much more comfortable with some nystatin suspension. When cups of tea were brought in and left for him to drink, he sometimes drank them. He slowly began to trust that he would not be forced into any action to which he did not agree and built up a rapport with one of the nurses through whom he finally agreed to have 4 hourly morphine for his pain and nystatin for his oral thrush. As he began to feel more comfortable he began to lose his suspicion and distrust. His partner was able to spend much time with him. Eventually the patient was able to make informed choices about his care, deal with a number of matters which, for him, were matters of unfinished business, renew and deepen relationships with the family. He died with a sense of achievement and at peace within himself. The end result was very rewarding for all concerned but the process involved a considerable amount of risk, and many painful encounters for staff.

Some patients are very skilled at manipulation; maybe they have had to spend most of their lives fighting to achieve good, or in 'beating the system'. Some patients' personalities are altered by HIV encephalopathy and some people are just manipulative. In such situations it is important that the team communicates, has a common approach which all members of the team understand and apply consistently, and that the boundaries are firmly and clearly explained to the patient. Freedom within boundaries can give a great sense of security and can still enable the patient to feel in control or to take responsibility. The boundaries and freedoms may require a certain amount of negotiation, but once agreed they should be seen as a contract that is binding to both parties, and treated as such. Again it is important that the contract is understood not only by the patient but by every member of the team.

This approach to care can be costly to staff who are used to a more directive or authoritarian approach, but it can also be immensely rewarding. In giving control back to the patient and placing responsibility where it belongs, with him, it can often also give him back a sense of identity and of worth, together with a restoration of his will to live.

> A patient, having lived for several weeks with considerable quality of life, said ten days before he died, 'The people here gave me back my will to live; this is the greatest gift that anyone can give to another human being'.

Reference

Wilkes, E., Harnett, G., Speed, D. *et al.* (1980). *Report of the working group on terminal care*. HMSO, London.

4   Nursing Issues

'The unique function of the nurse is to assist the individual, sick or well, in the performance of those activities, contributing to health or its recovery (or to a peaceful death) that he would perform unaided, if he had the necessary strength, will and knowledge'.

Henderson (1958)

The Wilkes (1980) report described terminal care as 'the provision of the very special support required by (terminally ill) patients and their families, and it is based, above all, on high quality nursing'.

Many people with AIDS are reminded of the reality of their situation every time they look into the mirror and see their wasted body or disfiguring lesions. To encourage these people to see value in life and carry on living takes considerable skill. Nurses need to utilise all their skills and ensure that their knowledge is adequately maintained in this developing area of care.

People with AIDS are often young people, facing a terminal illness, and many the same age as the nurses who are caring for them. These people may

— be emerging from the control of parents and/or educational and training establishments into a situation where they control and manage their lives, perhaps for the first time
— be living chaotic life styles, 'no one telling them what to do'
— as adults, have just found answers to conflicts affecting their lives, and have started 'really living' for the first time or
— have worked hard and moved up the promotional ladder to positions of responsibility or set up their own businesses, and are now at the peak of their career with 'the world as their oyster'.

Faced at this time, therefore, with the loss of the future they had hoped and planned for, it is not surprising that the majority of people with AIDS need to retain control over their lives.

The environment of care

People's homes vary enormously, but wherever they are and whatever they are like they usually offer security and safety. In their own home the occupant feels a sense of belonging, surrounded by 'their' things, things that are important to them and with which they are familiar. In their own home people can invite others in, keep others out, and be lone when they need to; they can eat, drink, wash, work and sleep when they choose to. People who do not live alone may not have the same ability to control their environment but will usually have a situation of negotiation and 'give and take'.

When care is given in a hospital or hospice *the environment should be made as comfortable and as home-like as possible.* Patients who are likely to be in a hospital or hospice for any length of time should be encouraged to bring in some small items from home, items that are important to him. The availability of books, magazines and tapes will help in providing a comfortable environment, as will an amenity fund from which flowers and extras can be bought for patients who have very little.

If patients are to have single rooms (consumer research at Mildmay indicates that this is clearly their preference) it is important that there are communal facilities where they can be with other people when they so wish. The privacy of their rooms should be respected and the patient consulted before visitors are allowed. It may be necessary to use 'please do not disturb' labels on doors to ensure that patients who need to rest are not disturbed by any of the team members without first consulting the nurse caring for that patient.

When a patient dies it is often appropriate that they are viewed in their own rooms, where 'good byes' can be said in a room that speaks of its resident, with familiar objects that speak of the living that took place in the midst of dying.

Flexibility

It is possible for patients to retain control over their lives whether they are being cared for in hospital, at home or in a hospice. In order to give patients control it is necessary for nurses to be given a greater degree of freedom and flexibility within the structure in which they work, so as not to be bound by routine and rigid time-tables. It will be necessary to ensure that managers understand the philosophy for nursing care so that inflexibility on their part does not restrict practice.

The structure in which care professionals work, the environment and inadequate resources may hinder the giving of control to patients. Lack of finance hinders every aspect of provision.

If there is only one bath, one shower, does this render routine essential?

Is service provision geared to patient needs or does the patient have to fit in with the system?

Dare you, can you change things in an established routine?

With the resistance of many carers to any change, and the directive attitude of many doctors and therapists, can you change to what may be a very different way of working?

What will help the nurse to make these changes?

— Acceptance of the need of most patients, not just those with AIDS to have control.
— Confidence in the nurse's own ability to cope with the outcome of giving control to patients.
— The need and the opportunity for nurses to examine and evaluate their practice.

The routine that involves learners in washing and getting up Mrs Smith, Mrs Brown and Mrs Jones before they go to coffee is still evident in some training hospitals. It is still possible to visit wards where the rules for nurses are 'Thou shalt not eat and drink on the ward'. What about when the best way to encourage a patient to eat is to take a meal with him? The hospitals and hospices which demonstrate flexibility and give control to patients are places where patients are living and positive attitudes are in evidence.

Relationships between the nurse, the patient and those close to him

Relationships with all patients should be based on mutual trust and acceptance and be confident and relaxed. Ensuring that one's knowledge and skills are adequate will enhance self confidence in the nurse, which in turn will inspire confidence in the patient and those close to him.

Primary nursing facilitates the establishment of good relationships between nurses and their patients and ensures continuity of care. It also allows nursing staff greater autonomy. Each patient has a specific nurse or nurses, with whom they can identify and work in partnership, so creating an environment suitable for making choices (Ersser and Tutton, 1990).

Rejection

Nurses usually find themselves in a situation of being needed and liked by their patients. This varies, of course, according to their area of care but most nurses enjoy the sharing in people's lives that nursing involves. The unresolved understandable anger that a few people with AIDS may have, at times presents itself in the need to reject others, including the nurse.

> A patient said to one nurse, 'If you think I find talking therapeutic, then you're wrong', and turned away every time she appeared. The nurse did not find the patient as hard to handle as her own feelings of being rejected, especially when talking was therapeutic for the patient with other nurses.

Some patients have not liked male nurses, female nurses or one nurse in particular. This problem is particularly apparent with patients with AIDS, perhaps because such patients feel that they are more able to make their own choices.

In dealing with rejection it is essential that nurses try to understand why the patient behaves in this way. It is important not to make assumptions but to establish facts. Nurses may need help and support (often from peers) to enable them to accept that the rejection is usually not personal but rejection of the system or displaced anger. If it is personal, the nurse needs to determine why someone responds to them in that way and, if possible, to remedy the situation. The nurse may need help and advice to see how he is perceived by others. Working together as a team and talking through difficulties with colleagues is often extremely helpful. In most instances the problems will be resolved, not by allowing the patient to make unreasonable demands, but by facing up to difficult problems with the patient and challenging when necessary. Giving patients choices may result in a patient refusing care from a particular nurse, and will present nurses with problems – problems that they must work through in order to be able to fulfil the duty of care they have to all patients.

Fear

Many nurses may be apprehensive about caring for people who are HIV antibody positive. Often it is not so much fear that they will become infected themselves, but that they might take 'something' home to their families and/or loved ones. The nurse's family may put pressure on the nurse, making it clear that they are not happy that he or she should expose him or herself, or them, to risk. These attitudes show that, although efforts have been made to educate and reassure, doubt, fear and misconception still exist. Television and newspaper reports often provide conflicting evidence, giving cause for concern. It is possible that, for many nurses, it is just 'fear of the unknown' that worries them, especially those nurses who have not yet cared for people with AIDS.

Relationships within the multiprofessional team

Whilst nurses have a key role in the terminal care of people with AIDS it is important that, by being 'jack of all trades', they do not exclude experts from other disciplines. It is often appropriate that the clinical nurse in charge is the coordinator of the multiprofessional team as she will be likely to have indepth information on all the patients (see also Chapter 3).

Principles of nursing care

In any care setting the principles of nursing care will be the same (see also Chapter 2).
— The unit of care is the patient and those important to him, be they family, partners or friends.

— Total nursing care is given to each patient as an appropriate response to their individual needs.
— The practice of nursing ensures continuity of care for the patient - this may involve visiting the patient prior to admission. Visits from community staff prior to discharge should be encouraged.
— Nurses encourage care to be self-directed by patients whenever possible. It may be necessary with some patients to provide a framework, agreed boundaries, within which a patient has control
— The nurse works in partnership with the patient toward the achievement of his aims and goals. The setting of short term achievable goals is a good motivating force.
— The emphasis should be on enhancing quality of life. It is important to make the most of every day and to make each day special.

Giving control where it belongs – to the patients – is often easier said than done. It involves

— accepting a challenge
— having the courage to change things
— being innovative – working out new ways of solving problems
— being willing to accept difficult outcomes
— taking risks.

But above all it involves re-inforcing the value that carers place on those they care for.

Infection control

If the care of people with AIDS is the nurses' responsibility, how are they going to deliver effective care to the patient while minimising the risk of infection to themselves and other patients?

Transmission of the virus may occur sexually, perinatally, by inoculation *in utero*, and rarely via breast milk. No other routes of spread are known. Therefore, the most important infection control measures are based on the prevention of inoculation accidents with used 'sharps', and the avoidance of frank contamination of skin and mucous membranes with blood and other body fluids. The following measures should be adopted.

1. Protective clothing – disposable plastic aprons and good quality disposable plastic or latex rubber gloves should be worn when the carer is exposed to blood and body fluids from any patient (including patients with HIV-related illness). This includes

— when dealing with bedpans and urinals
— when changing dressings
— when dealing with incontinence
— when collecting specimens
— when performing venepuncture or administering intravenous drugs and fluids

— when catheterising a patient and attending to sanitary needs
— when handling used instruments, clothes, linen or dressings soiled by body fluids
— when dealing with spillages of body fluids
— when touching non-intact skin.

2. Gloves and aprons should be discarded following contact with each patient or situation.

3. Masks and eye protection are only appropriate if caring for patients who have pulmonary involvement, are coughing excessively, or when assisting with invasive procedures during which splashing of body fluids may occur.

4. Any cuts or abrasions on the hands should be covered with water-proof dressings if contamination might occur.

5. Hands must be washed immediately with Hibiscrub or Betadine if contaminated with blood/body fluid secretions or excretions from any patient.

6. Care must be exercised when handling needles or other sharps. Needles and syringes should be disposable, and needles should not be resheathed or bent but should be placed immediately into a 'sharps' disposal bin.

7. Spillages of blood or body fluids should be covered with granules of sodium dichloroisocyanurate, such as Presept, left for a few minutes, and then carefully wiped up with disposable paper towels.

8. Members of staff who are immunodeficient/compromised either through illness or therapy, or suffering from exfoliative skin conditions should seek the advice of the occupational health department before nursing patients who are HIV positive.

The nurse must be aware of procedures which exist for the management of equipment, waste and linen which are potentially contaminated with opportunistic infective organisms. There may be local variations but there are certain general points. In the National Health Service in the UK, disposable contaminated articles and rubbish are placed in heavy duty yellow plastic bags, no other labelling being required. It is essential that needles and sharp ends of tubing should be removed and placed in a 'sharps' bin and not in the plastic bag. The yellow bags and 'sharps' bins are then incinerated. Linen soiled with blood and body fluids should be double bagged in red bags. The inner bag will be water soluble plastic and the outer red nylon. The red bags will be recognised as containing infected linen and no other labelling is required. In some areas a service is provided to patients in the community which involves the collection of infected, and the distribution of clean, linen.

Local policy will determine whether the nurse has a responsibility to decontaminate autoclavable and non-autoclavable instruments and equipment prior to return to CSSD. It will also determine how this is to be performed. Although HIV can be inactivated by most disinfectants, as people with AIDS frequently have several opportunist infections, disinfectants which are mycobacteriocidal, for example gluteraldehyde, are used for disinfecting all instruments which cannot be autoclaved. If not otherwise specified, used instruments should be bagged and labelled according to local policy and returned to CSSD. All rubbish not contaminated with blood and body fluids should be placed in the black plastic bags (non infected waste).

Home care

In many areas local authorities arrange for collection of waste for incineration and, as already stated, a few also have laundry services for infected linen.

Protective clothing in the form of plastic aprons and gloves should be available for staff and family/friends who assist with personal care, and the nurse should ensure that carers know when and when not to use them, and why.

Bins for sharps, and disinfectants (household bleach diluted 1:10 with water) and/or Presept granules or tablets should be kept in the house.

The household crockery and cutlery may be used by the patient; it is not necessary to keep separate utensils. Soiled linen can be washed satisfactorily on the hot cycle of a domestic washing machine. People with HIV can use the same toilet, bath and shower as the rest of the household and it will not need disinfecting after use.

It is NOT necessary to wear protective clothing of any sort for normal social contact with the patient, such as delivering food, post, counselling, chatting, pushing a wheelchair, shaking a patient's hand, or even giving him/her a hug.

In summary, the only precautions necessary (unless specifically stated) will be the use of gloves and aprons by those carers handling blood and body fluids. The same rule applies whether the patient is being cared for in hospital, in the community, or in a hospice.

The educational needs of nurses

In order to provide effective care nurses will need a comprehensive induction programme and on-going education and training to ensure a knowledge and understanding of related issues including
— the stigma of AIDS

— issues relating to altered body image and death and dying
— symptom control for people with AIDS
— listening and counselling skills
— issues relating to sexuality and drug addiction.

Support for nurses

It is recognised that nurses working in terminal care need considerable support, especially when coping with multiple bereavements. Wherever possible it is important that the structure within which they work is supportive in terms of the following.
— Manpower – adequate staffing levels with an appropriate skill mix
— Environment – absence of unnecessary rules and regulations
— Resources – adequate equipment to assist them to give high quality care
— Provision of appropriate training
— Commitment to staff development
— Availability and interest of the manager.
   In order to provide emotional support for staff in any setting it is essential to identify what it is that staff find to be helpful. Some nurses may find it helpful to talk to a counsellor on a one to one basis, others may find support groups of more value. Many will find their support by sharing with their peers, the friends they have made in their work setting. It is important not to overdo 'support', resulting in staff who find they are suddenly overwhelmed with problems they didn't even know they had.
   The comment made by Richard Wells in the foreword of Pratt (1989) provides a fitting conclusion to this chapter.

'The lack of a biomedical response to AIDS offers nursing the opportunity – probably for the first time – to prove what nursing is worth and to demonstrate that although the eventual outcome cannot be changed, the path to the outcome can be made less rigorous and more tolerable through nursing's interventions.'

References

Ersser, S. and Tutton, E. (Eds) (1990). *Primary Nursing in Perspective*. Scutari Press, London.
Henderson, V. (1958). *Basis Principles of Nursing Care*. International Council of Nurses, London.
Pratt, R. (1989). *AIDS: a Strategy for Nursing Care*, second edition. Edward Arnold, London.
Wilkes, E., Harnett, G., Speed, D. *et al.* (1980). *Report of the working group on terminal care*. HMSO, London.

5 Medical issues and dilemmas

Robert was a highly respected and much travelled business man in his 50s. When admitted to Mildmay for terminal care he was intermittently confused, very non-communicative, doubly incontinent, required 2 hourly turning, and refused to take food and drink for most of the time. His skin was very dry, he had seborrhoeic dermatitis, most noticeably on his face, and lymph oedema of the left leg with a large Kaposi's sarcoma (KS) lesion on the shin and a smaller one on the dorsal aspect of the foot. He had hepatomegaly, oral candidosis and dysphagia. Four months previously Robert had presented at a hospital with a dark purplish spreading lesion on the left shin, and complaining of tiredness. He had also noticed that his memory was not as good as usual, but had put this down to pressure at work and tiredness. Robert had noticed the lesion on his shin and one or two other smaller lesions elsewhere for several months beforehand but had not sought medical advice. He had also had intermittent diarrhoea from time to time and had lost some weight.

The biopsy of one of the purplish lesions showed that this was due to Kaposi's sarcoma and he was found to be HIV antibody positive. Further investigations revealed atypical mycobacteria in his stool and bone marrow – this was, on culture, found to be *Mycobacterium avium intracullulare* (MAI). A CT scan showed that he had mild cerebral atrophy. His KS lesions were treated with radiotherapy and he was started on anti-tuberculous treatment. As Robert had a history of herpes simplex infections, and one year prior to his diagnosis had had an episode of herpes zoster, he was also given Acyclovir prophylactically.

During the following three months Robert's condition deteriorated quickly. He continued to have problems with diarrhoea, vomiting and loss of weight. The KS lesions became more numerous and one in particular, on his left foot, caused swelling and discomfort in the foot with increased difficulty in walking. He became less and less mobile, increasingly depressed, more and more withdrawn and, at a later stage, intermittently confused. Robert gave his brother power of attorney.

When Robert was admitted to Mildmay, time was initially spent by the nursing team and the doctors in assessing his most obvious symptoms and dealing effectively with these. The nurses, in particular, spent time listening and just being with him and his partner. When he refused to take medication, this was discussed with him in detail by the doctor; his wishes to stop anti TB medication and Acyclovir were respected. However, with some negotiation he agreed to take those medications that had a direct effect on symptoms, including ketoconazole and nystatin oral suspension.

As his symptoms came under control, partly as a result of the care that he was receiving and partly as a result of stopping his anti-TB medication which had been contributing considerably to his nausea, Robert began to eat and drink small quantities again. As he regained a sense of control he also regained an interest in life, became less withdrawn and confused. Ten days after admission he took his first walk down to the lounge. During the following week he agreed to re-start his anti TB medication and, as his improvement continued, he requested radiotherapy for the KS on his left foot.

Robert took back his power of attorney and started holding business meetings from his room, sorting out his personal and business affairs. He was able to go home again to live independently with his partner (with whom he had lived for many years) for a short while before he was finally re-admitted for terminal care. In his final admission Robert once again required total nursing care, his HIV encephalopathy having progressed so that his symptoms were once again out of control. These were quickly brought under control and Robert died comfortably and with dignity several months after his initial admission.

Robert's story illustrates a number of medical dilemmas that are familiar to anyone dealing with life threatening illnesses. It also illustrates some issues which are directly related to AIDS. Direct symptom control details are dealt with in Chapter 6. This chapter considers some of the specific dilemmas and issues that are raised by the person with AIDS in the terminal care setting.

Is death synonymous with failure?

Doctors are generally trained to save life, or to prolong it, sometimes at great cost to the patient and to his carers. In an acute hospital setting death is often seen as a failure on the part of science and on the part of the doctors. The hospice movement has, in the past 20 years or so, taught us that death need not always be seen as a failure, or as an enemy. It may sometimes be a friend. When it is known, and accepted, that death is inevitable it is the quality of life that matters, not the quantity.

If Robert had died within the first week or two of his admission, perhaps his death could have been seen as a failure. With good symptom control and nursing care, and being given time, his interest in life was re-awakened. As he regained the sense of control he also regained his sense of identity and purpose. He was able to sort out his business affairs and leave his own personal affairs in good order. The quality of life for him and his partner included time together, first in the hospice unit and then at home.

As Robert's disease progressed, and in particular as the HIV encephalopathy became more obvious, his quality of life again changed for the worse. When re-admitted for terminal care he had had time to prepare himself and was now ready to face death. This time death was not a failure either by him or by the doctors, although it could be said to have been a failure of science in that a cure had not been found. However, an understanding of the principles of palliative medicine (a science in itself) had enabled the team to achieve comfort and dignity of the patient.

Prognosis and unpredictability

One of the most frequent questions a doctor is asked when dealing with a patient with a life threatening illness, is 'How long will it be, doctor? How long does he have?' This is always a difficult question to answer and the doctor who is foolhardy enough to give a definite statement will usually be proved wrong. This is particularly true for people with AIDS. AIDS is, as yet, a 'new' disease, with much to be learnt about the natural progress of the disease in its many different manifestations. The patients are often young, with a strong will to live and to remain in control, often persisting with active treatment until the very last. Patients in an apparently moribund state may recover sufficiently to require rehabilitation not only for themselves physically, but also emotionally for their carers, their families and their friends and partners.

In general, patients presenting with severe debility, weight loss and perhaps development of Kaposi's sarcoma lesions with a slow progression into AIDS survive for longer than patients who present with *Pneumocystis carinii* pneumonia (PCP) and other opportunistic infections. However, as Robert's story illustrates, this is not always the case.

Patient directed care

The advent of AIDS has challenged health care professionals to re-examine their attitudes to those who are in their care. People with AIDS have challenged health care professionals with their intelligent search for a greater understanding of their disease, their need to remain in control, their refusal to be treated as victims or to be 'fobbed off' by ambiguous answers or unclear explanations. The hospice movement and primary carers in the community have, in the past decade or two, led the way in revolutionising the approach to patients from that of 'the doctor knows best' to that of a partnership between the professional and the patient.

What does it mean in practice for the doctor to give control back to the patient and to be involved in patient directed care? It means that clear and honest information is given to patients, enabling them to make their own choices with appropriate guidance from the doctor, but never pressure. It means that the doctor has to accept the patient's choice. It means that the doctor's opinion will often be challenged: the doctor may often find that the patient knows more than the doctor does about his illness. It means that the doctor's opinion may be rejected and recommended medication or advice may not be taken. This can be difficult for the doctor to cope with, particularly when the doctor has been used to being in control and seen as an authority. However, if the doctor sees him or herself as a facilitator, enabler, information and advice giver then there need be no breakdown in the relationship or partnership.

When the patient is confused and demented who is in control? This issue must be discussed with other team members. The important question here is 'What would the patient have wished had he been able to make a decision?' This question can only be answered through a prior understanding and knowledge of the patient, and the best people to advise are the partner, the family or close friends. They should certainly be involved in decision making, particularly if the decision involves a major change in management policy.

It is all very well talking about, and seeking to put into practice, patient directed care when the patient wishes to have control, or is intelligent and able to understand the issues that are involved. It is a different matter to put this into practice when the patient does not wish to make decisions, or is unable to do so, or is manipulative, playing one member of the health care team off against another. A patient who wishes the doctor to make the decisions should have this wish respected until such time as they choose to take up that responsibility again.

Active versus palliative care

When is 'active therapy' in fact palliative? When treatments which are normally perceived as active are necessary (in terminal care) to maintain or improve quality of life, then that treatment can be termed palliative. Doctors should liaise closely with the referring consultants, and refer patients back to an acute centre for active therapy when a patient's condition deteriorates and he wishes to have active intervention.

Blood transfusions

The myelo-suppressive effects of Zidovudine, which is commonly used to slow down the replication of the virus and therefore the progress of the disease, often necessitate the giving of blood transfusions. Severe anaemias may develop, particularly in patients on high doses or who appear to be particularly sensitive. Other myelo-suppressive drugs, such as Gancyclovir may also contribute. It is clearly appropriate to give blood, when necessary, to someone who is having rehabilitative care, but how appropriate is it to give blood to someone who is terminally ill? In the author's experience the results of blood transfusions in patients who have shown signs of approaching the terminal phase have been disappointing, with very little change in physical energy and any appreciable change lasting, at most, for a couple of weeks. On occasion, there has been a subjective improvement, particularly in the patient's mental state. The decision as to whether or not to give a blood transfusion must be made according to the individual case, and must be made in consultation with the patient who may or may not feel that the trauma of having a blood transfusion is outweighed by the benefits.

Gancyclovir or Foscarnet infusions

Gancyclovir or Foscarnet infusions are given to prevent the progression of Cytomegalovirus (CMV) retinitis to total blindness. Even in the terminal weeks of life progression to blindness may be devastating for the patient, compounding his sense of isolation. It is therefore entirely appropriate, with the patient's cooperation and full understanding, to continue maintenance treatment. Gancyclovir and Foscarnet are usually given, through a central line which has been inserted under general or local anaesthesia in hospital, for the initial two to three weeks of treatment (see Chapter 6 for further details). Maintenance treatment is then continued, usually five times a week. If the maintenance therapy is stopped there is an increased risk of re-activation of CMV retinitis with further progression and damage to the eye. When treatment has already been instituted in hospital and maintenance therapy is being given as a matter of course, clearly these treatments should be continued. However, difficult decisions may have to be faced when a patient who may only have weeks to live develops CMV retinitis for the first time.

A patient, who on many occasions told the doctor and the nurses that he wished to die and that no active intervention should be made, developed CMR retinitis with what appeared to be only weeks to live. He was already extremely cachetic and weak and could not face further acute treatment, with the transferal to an acute centre, frequent blood tests and daily infusions. His mother agreed with him. However, as his vision deteriorated and he lingered longer than expected, some of the staff found this decision extremely difficult to live with although the patient seemed undistressed. He died three weeks later. His gentle acceptance and quiet withdrawal as death approached made it clear that he was content with his decision, but the difficulty the staff had to face was the uncertainty of his total understanding of the issues involved when he had made the decision as he was also intermittently confused. The question sometimes has to be asked 'Who would we be treating – the patient, or ourselves and our anxiety?'

Foscarnet is frequently given during the initial treatment phase as a continuous infusion over 24 hours for 3 weeks, followed by maintenance therapy given 5 times a week over 4 to 8 hours. This kind of therapy is very restrictive for the patient and, together with the frequent blood tests that are required to monitor the nephrotoxic effect, may detract considerably from the possible quality of life that is available to the patient. What constitutes quality of life for one patient may be quite different for another and decisions must be made with each individual, and must be regularly reviewed.

Both Gancyclovir and Foscarnet infusions can be given in the home, provided that either the patient is able to give the infusions himself, or the community nurses are able to take on this task. Patients can be taught to give their own infusions, however this may not be possible for patients developing encephalopathy or other neurological problems, or as their illness progresses and they become weaker.

A patient whose prognosis was extremely uncertain but who had been fairly stable for some months opted for referral from the hospice unit back to his acute centre for insertion of the Hickman line, followed by a return to the hospice for the continuation of the initial treatment and then maintenance therapy. He eventually learnt to give his own infusion and was able to return home for some months. (See p. 52)

If home treatment is not possible, a Day Centre may enable the patient to have the treatment but still live at home.

Total parenteral nutrition (TPN)

Maintenance of total nutrition via a central line is an increasingly popular option for patients suffering from the debilitating effects of persistent severe diarrhoea caused by cryptosporidiosis, together with the nausea and vomiting that often accompanies it. Both the diarrhoea and the vomiting are very resistant to treatment and control may be very difficult to achieve without unacceptable side effects (see also Chapter 6). High standards of aseptic technique are required to prevent infection, regular blood tests once or twice weekly are needed to ensure correct electrolyte and nutritional balance, and close liaison is required between the doctor, the dietitian, the pharmacist who makes up the mixture, and the laboratory services. For the patient with oesophageal KS or intractable vomiting and diarrhoea, but whose prognosis is otherwise reasonably good, this may be a viable option. It then becomes a life-line, and the question arises as to when this life-line should be cut. This may be an enormously difficult question for both the patient and his family to cope with and it may, indeed, never be faced, either by them or by the doctors and nurses involved. Since it is the nurses who generally set up the TPN and who are more intimately involved with the patient they may well be the first to ask the question; and they may be the best people to begin the discussion with the patient or the family.

Total parental nutrition can, of course, be given at home or in the community, provided there is someone trained and able to maintain the high aseptic standards that are required in giving the daily infusion. The general practitioner or home care team and dietitian will have to liaise closely with laboratory services and pharmacists to ensure successful continuation of this therapy, which requires a high level of commitment by all.

Investigations

Some investigations involve quite traumatic procedures. In the case of the patient who is having rehabilitative or convalescent care and is not yet obviously terminally ill, it is clear that any sudden deterioration or change should be investigated, and decisions have to be made about where these investigations should take place. However, when somebody has entered the terminal phase of the illness the question should be asked, 'Who will benefit from this investigation? What change in management will be indicated by the result of the investigation?' In other words, if the result of any investigation is likely to substantially alter the management, then it is appropriate for the investigation to be done. However, if the investigation is merely for academic satisfaction then it may be quite inappropriate to subject either the patient or his family to the trauma involved in taking blood tests, performing lumbar punctures etc. Of course it is important to add to the total knowledge that we have about AIDS, but this need has to be balanced against the rights and needs of the patient.

Protection for the doctor and other health care professionals

All body fluids should be treated with respect, whether they are known or not to come from someone who is HIV positive. Gloves should be worn by anyone coming into contact with body fluids or at risk of doing so, and a plastic apron worn to protect clothes. Gloves should also be worn by anyone taking blood, and of course whenever intravenous injections or infusions are set up. These same standards should ideally be applied wherever care is being given, not only to people known to have AIDS but to all categories of patients, and all blood should be treated as potentially infected, either with Hepatitis B or HIV. Further information on infection control is given on pp. 32–33.

Radiotherapy and chemotherapy

In the terminal phases of advanced AIDS, radiotherapy may be appropriate to provide palliation for a severely swollen limb as a result of KS, and chemotherapy may reduce oesophageal obstruction caused by KS and may also reduce pain associated with swallowing. However, again side effects may outweigh the benefits and decisions may have to be made regarding the continuation of or the stopping of therapy. These decisions cannot be arrived at without discussion of all the available options and possible outcomes.

> A patient admitted for terminal care with KS involving most of the lower lobe of the right lung regained his determination and will to live to such an extent that he was prepared to undergo radiotherapy to his lung and to several skin lesions to a total of 13 treatments. Each of these involved an ambulance trip across London to the radiotherapy centre in the referring hospital. The patient was warned that the prognosis for someone with KS lung was usually a matter of weeks and at best with radiotherapy a few months, at most six or seven. Two and a half months after admission he was discharged to sheltered accommodation where he lived with his partner with considerable quality of life for a further six months.

For this patient the benefits of treatment far outweighed the disadvantages, but for others it does not.

> A patient with the same problem as mentioned above opted to have no active intervention, but accepted symptom control measures which made him very comfortable and enabled him to live the final three or four weeks of his life with great zest and enjoyment, in spite of the increasing dyspnoea and general weakness. He preferred to conserve his energies for settling his affairs, being reconciled with his family, and meeting Her Royal Highness, The Princess of Wales when she visited the hospice unit.

When death approaches

In most cases it is clear to all involved with a patient that he is deteriorating. However, as has already been said, it is extremely risky to prognosticate as patients often have a very strong will and determination to live. In the author's experience some patients have clung on to their regular daily dosages of Zidovudine until the day they died; some, as illustrated by the case histories given here, have confounded all prognostications, recovered against all odds and have been able to go home, albeit for a short while. However, there comes a time when it is evident that the patient is entering the terminal phase and probably has only a few days to live – when the patient has become increasingly weak and immobile, is less interested in food and drink, spends much of the day sleeping or drowsy, and may have developed signs of an early broncho-pneumonia. The question then arises, 'Who do you tell and how much?' The patient is usually aware and may or may not wish to speak about his situation. The partner and family or close friends are anxious to know 'How long?' and 'What will happen?' It should never be acceptable to say there is nothing more that can be done, to say that those responsible for providing care have given up. *There is always something more that can be done to ensure the patient's comfort and ease from distress.*

The family need to be aware that the patient may linger for several days longer than expected. During this time the family may wish to see the doctor frequently and will certainly require a great deal of support and comfort from the nursing and other staff. The family require reassurance that the patient will not suffer; with good symptom control this assurance can be given with confidence.

How much do you tell? The answer to this question depends to some extent on your relationship with the family and friends and with the patient. It is important that all members of the team know what is being said and discussed and that those who are close to the patient are not given conflicting information. It is also sometimes important to spare them from unnecessarily distressing details.

A patient developed CMV retinitis within days of death. It was obvious to the hospice staff that the patient was becoming blind, but they felt that it was an unnecessarily distressing detail with which to burden the mother, especially as the patient seemed not to be distressed.

The doctor's role in terminal care

Within the multiprofessional team the doctor must work in close cooperation with the nursing team, listening to them as well as to the patient and those who are close to him. As has already been suggested, the nurses provide the most intimate care and spend the longest time with the patient, so are in an ideal position to observe and understand the needs of the patient. The doctor is one member of the full multiprofessional team and must also liaise closely with chaplains, physiotherapists, occupational therapists and counsellors, as well as social workers or others involved. He or she must also maintain contact with and liaise with consultants and other doctors who have been involved in the patient's care so that appropriate and coordinated care is given on a continuing basis. During the final few days it is the doctor's duty to monitor closely the results of symptom control measures, together with the nurses involved and then to certify death when this occurs.

After death the family continues to require support, but the doctor's role here is clearly to deal with such practical matters such as the death certificate, cremation form and autopsies where appropriate as quickly and as efficiently as possible. It is important to have thought through the whole issue of what goes on the death certificate before the actual time comes when the certificate has to be written. The word 'AIDS' on a death certificate can cause a tremendous amount of trauma to the family, as death certificates are not private property and are available for inspection by a number of bodies. It is acceptable to write only the immediate and obvious cause of death, such as broncho-pneumonia or viral encephalitis with associated causes of death such as CMV infection, mycobacterial disease etc., on the death certificate. Box B, offering further information, is ticked on the form, and this may be accompanied by a covering and confidential letter stating that the patient had the diagnosis of AIDS. The cremation forms have the same wording as the death certificate.

The educational needs of the doctor

Doctors who are involved in terminal and continuing care for people with AIDS are privileged to share in the darkness (see Dr Sheila Cassidy's (1988) book, *Sharing the Darkness*), but also in some of the trials, and even joys, that the patient and those close to him will be going through. It is, inevitably, a time of deep sadness and trauma for all involved. All those involved in the patient's care will be looking to the doctor for guidance and for information about the cause of the disease, about its management, about the prognosis, and for symptom control. It is vitally important that the doctor is fully aware of the progress of the disease. It is also very important that doctors keep up to date with current knowledge, maintain close contacts with colleagues and other sources of information about the current state of research into new drugs, vaccines and other therapies. If doctors do not have the knowledge themselves, they should at least know where to turn for information and advice.

Support for doctors

Doctors do not only need to keep up to date clinically. Anyone involved in the care of people with life threatening illnesses will be aware that he or she will frequently face deep searching questions, and difficult dilemmas. Doctors may find that their beliefs or world views are seriously challenged, and experience the emotional draining that comes with multiple bereavement. It is therefore important that doctors recognise their own needs in terms of support. This support may be available through the multiprofessional team, through colleagues, family or other support networks such as church or friends. Individuals will have their own support network. If doctors are to continue to provide effective support to the patients and their families during this special, but very traumatic, time and afterwards, they must ensure that they have support for themselves.

6 Symptom control and common medical problems

'...meticulous attention to detail can lead to appropriate and effective treatment to the end of a patient's life. This transforms his experience, and the memories of his family.'

Dame Cicely Saunders in Twycross and Lack (1990) '

The above quotation from Dame Cicely Saunders' Foreword to the well known book *Therapeutics in Terminal Cancer* is equally true for the care of patients with advanced AIDS. A conversation overheard in the street, where one woman was saying to another 'The doctor said there was nothing more they could do for him...' is still sadly the experience of many people. In terms of a cure, it is of course true that there comes a time when nothing more can be done to achieve a cure, or to prolong life with quality. However, it is never true that nothing more can be done to make a patient more comfortable.

This chapter is set in the context of a book which seeks throughout to deal with the needs of the whole person. Good medical management and symptom control is only one aspect of the whole. However, it is an aspect of care which may profoundly affect the experience of the patient, and the memories with which the partners, families or friends have to live for many years to follow. Their memories may also profoundly affect their own attitudes to facing issues of death and dying.

A patient with severe peripheral neuropathy, which was proving difficult to control, was found, on probing more deeply, to have vivid memories of his father's problems with severe diabetic neuropathy and eventual bilateral above knee amputations prior to his death. These memories were very frightening and undoubtedly affected his own reaction to the peripheral neuropathy that he was experiencing.

Of necessity, this chapter must be brief in giving only an overview of the way in which advanced AIDS presents in the terminal care situation, with a description of the common symptoms encountered and guidelines for dealing with them, and some comments about common medical problems which may present management difficulties. It is based on the experience gained since February 1988 when Mildmay opened its hospice unit for people with AIDS. It was the first such unit in Europe and therefore had no model to follow. The principles of palliative care in cancer gave us our basic guide-lines but much of our learning as a team was experiential. We learned from and with each other, but most of all we learnt from and with our patients.

Good symptom control in advanced AIDS depends on the following:

Attention to detail   It is important to invest time to examine the patient in detail and to listen carefully to his description of his problems and symptoms. Careful assessment of the degree to which a symptom is felt should also be made; this is particularly relevant in dealing with a symptom such as pain where good control will depend on meticulous monitoring of the response to therapy. It is important to bear in mind that significant changes can take place very rapidly in a patient with AIDS and that the doctor's perception of a problem may differ considerably from that of the patient himself.

Good *liaison* and *communication* between nurses and doctors. Nurses are the people who spend most time with the patient, and are involved in many intimate procedures which mean that they are in an excellent position to observe and monitor symptoms and the result of medication. Many nurses are skilled listeners and observers, and often the patients will discuss details with the nurses that they would not talk about with the doctor.

A good *knowledge* and *understanding* of:
— AIDS and its presentation in the advanced stages of the disease
— the drugs commonly used in the treatment of AIDS and related problems
— the therapeutic principles of palliative medicine e.g. pain control.

Many good books have been written about the basic principles of terminal care in cancer and other life threatening illnesses to which reference should also be made. This chapter will deal with the differences encountered in caring for someone with AIDS, although there are, of course, some overlapping areas of care which will also be dealt with briefly where appropriate. (See the Introduction for a list of differences.)

The patient

Patients with AIDS cannot and should not be categorised and grouped. Nor is it possible to describe any one particular type of patient. Chapter 2 described, in the authors' experience, some of the main differences encountered in patients. However, it must be remembered that this experience is limited by location in the West and in a large cosmopolitan capital city. It is, nevertheless, true to say that people with AIDS will,

n the main, be young people, many of them in what should be the
prime of their lives. The majority of people with AIDS, in the West,
apart from children or people with haemophilia, will be in the age range
of 20–49 years.

Multiple diagnoses and inevitable polypharmacy

All patients with AIDS will have a number of co-existing diagnoses,
many of which will be opportunistic infections for which the patient
will be receiving treatment for active infections, maintenance therapy
for control of persisting problems, or prophylaxis to prevent recurrence
of opportunistic infections.

Many patients will also require drugs related specifically to symptom
control. Some symptoms, for example nausea and vomiting, might be
directly related to the drugs the patient is taking. Other symptoms such
as pain or parathesiae, dysphagia, or diarrhoea might be due to the
effects of the HIV virus itself, or of opportunistic infections. Although
the number of drugs that a patient may be taking might be rationalised,
and in some cases reduced, the doctor is often forced into practising
polypharmacy in trying to control or prevent the recurrence of distressing or painful conditions such as herpes simplex or a life-threat-
ening condition such as cerebral toxoplasmosis or *Pneumocystis carinii*
pneumonia (PCP). The time will inevitably come when it is appropriate
to stop prophylactic treatment; this is obvious when the patient has
become unconscious or is no longer able to take oral medications, but
not so obvious when the patient is still conscious and anxious about
the possible onset, for example, of PCP or dementia. Such decisions
have to be made in discussions with the patient, with where possible
explanation of the likely outcomes. Some patients for example, find
acyclovir difficult to swallow, and although there are few side effects,
patients will often opt to stop this drug. Septrin is another tablet that
many dislike taking. Most of the anti-tuberculous drugs are also difficult
to take and cause nausea and vomiting; many patients improve sub-
jectively on stopping these medications. Robert's story at the beginning
of Chapter 5 illustrates a number of these points.

Common conditions and infections found in AIDS

This section does not attempt or pretend to be an exhaustive introduction to clinical aspects of AIDS. It is intended to provide the general
practitioner, hospice doctor, or other health care professional involved
with a terminally ill AIDS patient, with a brief introduction to the
conditions and infections most likely to be encountered. Where appropriate the prognostic significance of certain conditions is indicated and
information on available treatment options given. Readers who wish
to know more about AIDS and its many complex manifestations, its

immunology and epidemiology should refer to the many good tex
books and journals that are available (see Further reading).

Common opportunistic infections

Pneumocystis carinii pneumonia *(PCP)*

PCP is caused by a protozoan which exists in cyst or trophozoite form
within pulmonary alveoli. A definitive diagnosis of PCP can only b
made upon finding the organisms on microscopy (through bronch
alveolar lavage with production of sputum or on bronchoscopy). In th
terminal care situation neither of these diagnostic investigations ar
likely to be appropriate. PCP is characterised by a persistent dry cough
with persistent or increasing dyspnoea and, quite frequently, very fev
clinical signs in the chest. PCP is often associated with Cytomegal
virus (CMV) infections, but there are also a number of other causes o
pneumonias and pulmonary problems such as Kaposi's sarcoma. (Se
Table 13, pp. 72–76 for treatment and prophylaxis of PCP.)

   In someone whose general condition is fairly good and who is anxiou
to continue with active treatment, investigations to establish the exac
cause of pulmonary problems are appropriate, but in the terminally il
patient such investigations may be of little significance in terms of actua
management, and the patient should not be subjected to unnecessar
distress. Clinical judgement as to the pertinence of pursuing activ
treatment in someone who has developed a chest infection in fa
advanced AIDS must depend on the patient himself and what he wishes
as well as on his general condition at the time and the potential fo
quality of life which still exists. It may be appropriate in some situation
to offer antibiotic therapy.

Cytomegalovirus (CMV)

CMV is a member of the herpes group of viruses and is widely sprea
through the general population with particularly high prevalence rate
in densely populated areas. Congenital CMV infections may caus
serious neurological problems but acquired infection in adults onl
rarely cause serious illness. However in AIDS, where HIV causes
deficiency in cell mediated immunity, CMV infections are associate
with disseminated disease affecting many organs. CMV is commonl
associated with PCP and may also cause encephalitis, colitis or oeso
phagitis. However the most serious effect is on the retina where i
causes retinitis which, if left untreated, may progress rapidly to tota
blindness. Patients admitted for long term terminal care should b
examined every few weeks for signs of CMV retinitis as it may initiall
be asymptomatic. The patient may complain simply of blurring of visio
or have noticed recent problems with peripheral vision. Examination o
the fundi will reveal soft exudates (cotton wool spots) or haemorrhage
and should be immediately referred for ophthalmological opinion an

reatment. It is often unilateral and even if only partial vision is possible n one eye, the other eye may be spared by treatment and maintenance herapy (Gancyclovir or Foscarnet by infusion via a central or Hickman ine, usually 5 days per week). CMV oesophagitis, colitis and hepatitis re less common. CMV oesophagitis causes severe burning retro-sternal ɔain with dysphagia, and CMV colitis causes a watery diarrhoea which may be profuse, and occasionally causes fresh bleeding. It may be ɩccompanied by abdominal pain and distension; occasionally per-ɔration of the bowel may occur. There may be fever and, inevitably, veight loss. Foscarnet or Gancyclovir infusions may be successful in educing the volume of diarrhoea and in improving the general con-lition of the patient.

Toxoplasmosis

This is caused by the protozoan *Toxomplasma gondii* which infects ɩumans after ingestions of cysts in infected meat or cat faeces. Released ʻrom the cysts in the gastro-intestinal tract, the active tachyzoites enter he blood stream via the gastric mucosa and spread to all tissues in the ɔody, but particularly to the brain, although disseminated infection may affect the heart, liver, lungs and spleen were abscesses may form. Focal neurological problems are the commonest signs of development. The diagnosis is made by CT or MRI scan and active treatment insti-ʇuted, although brain biopsy is required for definitive diagnosis. Most ɔatients remain on prophylaxis following initial treatment.

In the terminally ill patient toxoplasmosis may be reactivated and lisseminated in spite of prophylaxis, or as a result of stopping this when ʇhe patient is no longer able or willing to take medication. Prophylaxis ɩs usually in the form of Fansidar (a combination of Pyrimethamine ɩnd Sulphadoxine), one or two tablets daily (see also Table 13, ɔp. 72–76). These may also be given separately, together with folinic ɩcid (15 mg od), as the folic acid levels are reduced by these drugs ʇherefore causing megaloblastic anaemia.

Mycobacterial disease

Mycobacterial disease in general is more common in patients with AIDS than in other patients. *Mycobacterial tuberculosis* causes typical pulmonary disease which may or may not be resistant to treatment, depending on geographical area and resistance patterns. Atypical myco-bacteria are frequently resistant to most conventional drug regimes. MAI is a complex of 2 strains, *Mycobacterium avium* and *Myco-bacterium intracellulare* and has been found in approximately 50 per cent of AIDS patients at post mortem. Other atypical mycobacteria are found in AIDS, for example *M. xenopi* and *M. kanasaii*. MAI is the most common form found in the UK and usually causes disseminated disease affecting the gut, bone marrow, liver, lung, spleen, adrenal glands, brain, lymph nodes and kidney. Diagnosis is made by finding acid fast bacilli and culturing appropriate samples. Treatment is with anti-tuberculous medication such as a combination of, for example, Rifabutin, ethambutol, pyrazinamide, and isoniazid. These commonly cause side effects such as nausea and vomiting and, as the patient's general condition deteriorates, some patients may opt to stop treatment. As MAI is highly resistant this would seem appropriate when trying to enhance quality of life (unless there is a risk to other patients from open infection). It is possible that the alleviation of anorexia and nausea achieved by stopping these medications can lead to an improvement in the general condition of the patient. The patient may be able to resume medication at a later stage, as is illustrated by Robert's story (p. 36).

On laparotomy, prior to admission, a patient was found to have disseminated abdominal tuberculosis and opted to stop all anti-tuberculous medication. Soon after admission for terminal care he developed symptoms and signs of an acute abdomen. He chose to remain at the hospice, and was started on 8 mg of Dexamethasone daily which was gradually reduced over a period of weeks to 1 mg daily. He recovered rapidly from his acute abdomen and his general condition improved so that over a period of time he was able to go home every weekend and after several months went home to stay with his parents where he lived until he died almost a year after his initial admission. The patient continued to refuse anti-tuberculous medication, and was maintained throughout on either 0.5 or 1 mg of Dexamethasone. Attempts at stopping this always resulted in a recurrence of symptoms and a deterioration in his general well-being. Six months prior to his death he also developed CMV retinitis, and did opt to have a Hickman line inserted and intra-venous Gancyclovir therapy. He retained the vision of one eye but lost most effective vision in the other. The patient eventually succumbed to disseminated Mycobacterial disease.

Cryptosporidial and other diarrhoeas

Cryptosporidium muris is a parasite which causes damage to the gastro intestinal mucosa, with fusion of villi and production of a profuse watery diarrhoea, sometimes amounting to 8 to 10 litres per day. It is usually accompanied by abdominal pain, loud borborygmi and flatulence, severe general malaise and loss of weight, with malabsorption. There may be fever, and in some patients nausea and vomiting are a prominent feature. Even when the cryptosporidiosis has been successfully treated, which is frequently not possible, the patient may be left with permanent mucosal damage leading to diarrhoea and continued malabsorption. A very large number of drugs have been tried in an attempt to treat this infection, but none with any significant degree of success although occasional individuals have responded to treatment. In the terminal care situation diarrhoea should be controlled as far as possible with oral rehydration fluid, anti-diarrhoeal and anti-emetic drugs, as well as, where possible, treatment of the cause. In cryptosporidiosis it is usually effective to start with loperamide 4–8 mg qds (up to maximum of 32 mg in 24 hours—above the usual recommended dose, but safe with no CNS effects). The addition of Isphaghula in the form of Fybogel twice or three times daily will thicken the stool and an antispasmodic such as buscopan (hyoscine butyl bromide may also help. Constipation is not likely to occur, even with regular medication, and for some patients it is necessary to use opiates. Once it has been decided to use opiate medication, the appropriate dosage should be titrated in the normal way using 4 hourly morphine or diamorphine initially orally, until some success in controlling the diarrhoea has been achieved, then changing to 12 hourly dosages of sustained release morphine sulphate tablets for convenience. In a patient who has intractable vomiting, diamorphine in a syringe driver may be very effective in combination with an anti-emetic such as metoclopramide, haloperidol or, in severe cases, methotrimeprazine. It is not always possible to prevent the diarrhoea completely; however it has been possible to reduce the frequency of diarrhoea from perhaps 10, 12 or more times to 3 or 4 times in 24 hours, sometimes down to 1 or 2. Stool volumes may continue to be large even at this frequency.

It is becoming more common to give total parenteral nutrition through a Hickman/central line to patients with the severe weight loss and wasting that is associated with this kind of diarrhoea. TPN is also given to patients with oesophageal obstruction as a result of KS or lymphoma. Weekly or twice weekly blood tests are necessary to ensure electrolyte and nutritional balance, and close liaison is required between doctors, the dietitian, the pharmacist and the laboratory services. Meticulous aseptic techniques must be maintained by those who are involved in setting up the daily TPN (usually the nurses but patients may also learn to do this themselves to maintain independence – see also Chapter 5).

Table 1 suggests the recommended therapy for the control of nausea, vomiting and diarrhoea in cryptosporidiosis. Other pathological organisms which cause diarrhoea should be treated appropriately when isolated, with normal symptom control and fluid replacement for the diarrhoea.

Candida albicans

Candida albicans is the most common cause of mouth problems in HIV disease. It manifests itself through inflammation and soreness with the typical white plaques of oral thrush which, when severe, may coat the tongue, the hard and soft palate, the mucosal lining and gums and may also spread into the pharynx. *Candida albicans* may affect the whole of the gastro-intestinal tract, and commonly also affects the oesophagus. The symptoms vary from dryness or soreness of the mouth to severe retro-sternal discomfort and dysphagia. Until recently ketoconazole

Table 1   Control of nausea, vomiting and diarrhoea in cryptosporidiosis.

Symptom	Recommended therapy
Nausea/vomiting	Metoclopramide* PO/IM 10–20 mg tds Cyclizine PO/IM/PR 25–50 mg tds Haloperidol* PO/s–c 0·5–5 mg bd possibly Nabilone PO 1–2 mg bd
Intractable vomiting	*via syringe driver if necessary; also methotrimeprazine starting with 25–50 mg over 12 hours Sometimes required in combination
Diarrhoea	Loperamide 4–8 mg qds (max. 32 mg in 24 hours) Fybogel 1–3 sachets daily
Intractable diarrhoea	Morphine/diamorphine PO or s–c by syringe driver (titrate dose in usual way)

Higher dosages may be necessary.
Persistent nausea or diarrhoea should not be treated on a prn basis.

has been the drug of choice for treatment and prophylaxis. The drugs itraconazole and fluconazole, both of which are less hepatotoxic and cause fewer side effects, have now become more popular. As they can also be given as a single oral daily dose they are easier to take. When a patient is unable to take oral medication it is usually possible to continue with nystatin suspension, which should be given regularly every 2 to 4 hours and held in the mouth for as long as possible. In immuno-compromised patients higher doses may be required than those recommended by the manufacturers (Meunier-Carpenter, 1984). Some people dislike the taste and prefer to suck pastilles of nystatin or amphotericin lozenges. However, these do tend to make the mouth feel dry and furred up and, in someone who is becoming dehydrated as a result of reduced oral in-take, this can be a problem. Good oral hygiene with regular chlorhexidine mouth washes or gel may be as important as medication. Table 2 indicates other common oral conditions with which the AIDS patient may present.

Herpes infections

Herpes simplex infections are very common and cause oral or oeso-phageal ulceration, or ano-rectal and genital problems with ulceration and pain (see Table 3). Oral and oesophageal ulceration has been dealt with above; ano-rectal and genital *Herpes simplex* infections are particularly common in homosexual patients. In ano-rectal herpes infec-tion, defaecation is usually very painful with severe tenesmus. Treat-

Table 2 Common oral conditions, other than *Candida albicans*.

Condition	Treatment/comment
Hairy leucoplakia (white adherent patches on sides of tongue associated with Epstein-Barr virus)	Seldom causes problems, therefore treatment is not usually necessary
Gingivitis and dental abscesses	Dental advice and good oral hygiene
Herpes simplex	
stomatitis	Acyclovir 200–400 mg × 5 per day
oesophageal ulceration	Acyclovir IV
CMV infection; oral or oesophageal ulceration	May respond to IV DHPG or Foscarnet
Aphthous ulceration	Hydrocortisone 2·5 mg lozenges Betamethasone 0·1 mg pellets (both applied directly to the ulcer) Benzydamine (Difflam) mouthwash; if very painful and extensive – Thalidomide 50–100 mg daily

ments of 400 mg of acyclovir 5 times daily for 5 days may be very effective in dealing both with the infection and the pain. After cleaning with normal saline, acyclovir cream applied to the peri-anal area or to ulcers on the penis or scrotum, will ease the symptoms and promote healing.

Herpes zoster, causing chickenpox or shingles, is said to occur in up to 50 per cent of patients with HIV disease. Shingles is a common sign of immuno-suppression and in HIV disease may present in more than one dermatome, or may recur. Post-herpetic neuralgia may persist and require treatment with, for example, carbamazepine. There is a risk of *Herpes zoster* meningitis and patients are usually given acyclovir prophyclactically.

Cryptococcal meningitis

Cryptococcal meningitis is caused by the yeast *Cryptococcus neoformans*. It is treated with intravenous amphotericin B with or without oral or intravenous flucytosine. In the terminal care setting the decision about whether or not to investigate and actively treat signs of meningitis will depend on the patient's general condition, other co-existing problems and any known wishes as to active intervention. If treatment is started and tolerated it is usually necessary to continue for several weeks; recurrence is common and long term prophylactic anti-fungal treatment may be necessary although not very effective (e.g. itra-

Table 3   Herpes infections.

Condition	Treatment
Herpes simplex*	
Stomatitis	Acyclovir 200–400 mg × 5 per day
Oesophageal ulcer	IV acyclovir
Ano-rectal herpes simplex (may cause severe tenesmus)	Acyclovir 200–400 mg × 5 per day × 5 days
	Acyclovir cream × 5 per day
Herpes simplex on penis or	Acyclovir 200–400 mg × 5 per day × 5 days
scrotum	Acyclovir cream × 5 per day
Herpes zoster*	
Chickenpox or shingles in one or more dermatomes	Acyclovir 800 mg × 5 per day × 7 days
Post herpetic neuralgia	Carbamazepine, also clonazepam in some cases
Ophthalmic or neurological complications	IV acyclovir and specialist supervision

* Risk of meningitis or encephalitis if left untreated or not taking prophylaxis following first infection.

conazole or fluconazole), or amphotericin B given as a daily intravenous infusion.

Progressive multifocal leuco-encephalopathy (PML)

PML is a sub-acute demyelinating disease of the central nervous system and is caused by the papova virus. It has been described in a number of conditions in which cell mediated immunity is impaired. PML causes multiple lesions in the white matter of the cerebrum causing focal neurological signs. Lesions may also occur in the brain stem and cerebellum. It is rapidly progressive and no treatment has been found to be effective. Signs and symptoms of the disease may be focal neurological problems, ataxia, mental deterioration and even cortical blindness and paralysis. The prognosis is often poor, with death occurring usually within weeks or months after diagnosis (by CT scan and/or brain biopsy). HIV infection may also cause leuco-encephalopathy, often producing a similar picture.

HIV encephalopathy and other neurological problems in HIV disease

HIV is known to be neurotropic. There is some evidence to suggest that defective methylation with demyelination may play a part in the neurological damage caused by HIV infection. Post mortem findings have been surveyed and indicated that a very high proportion of people

Table 4 Neurological conditions in HIV disease (from Youle *et al.*, 1988, *AIDS: Therapeutics in HIV Disease*. Churchill Livingstone).

Human immunodeficiency virus	
Seroconversion illness	Encephalitis
	Meningitis
	Myelitis
	Nerve palsies
Chronic manifestations	Encephalopathy
	Recurrent meningitis
	Vacuolar myelopathy
	Peripheral neuropathy
	Autonomic neuropathy
Other infections	
Toxoplasma gondii	Cerebral abscesses
Cytomegalovirus	Retinitis, encephalitis
Cryptococcus neoformans	Meningitis
Papova virus	Progressive multifocal leucoencephalopathy (PML)
Mycobacterium tuberculosis	Meningitis, cerebral abscesses
Herpes zoster	Meningitis, Ramsey–Hunt syndrome
Candida albicans	Cerebral abscesses
Nocardia asteroides	Cerebral abscesses
Tumours	
Primary CNS lymphoma	Space occupying lesion

with HIV disease develop minor or major neurological problems. Lantos *et al.* (1989) reported that, in a survey, nearly 90 per cent of the patients reviewed had cerebral abnormalities. These findings confirm those of the surveys done in America where it is commonly referred to as AIDS dementia complex (ADC) (Gabuzda and Hirch, 1987). This is an extremely complex subject and the reader is referred to the relevant text books and journals for further information. In summary, and for the purposes of differential diagnosis, Table 4 is reproduced with kind permission of Michael Youle *et al.* (1988).

HIV encephalopathy

Early minor signs of HIV encephalopathy (see Table 5) may present in a number of patients with AIDS. The increasing expertise in the treatment of acute opportunistic infections is now enabling people with AIDS to survive far longer, but it does mean that increasing numbers will develop the more advanced signs of HIV encephalopathy. It is important to differentiate between HIV encephalopathy and other causes with similar signs and symptoms, for example toxoplasmosis, neuro-syphillis, or drug induced confusion, as these may be treatable. It is also important to remember that any infection or febrile condition may cause confusion, as may hypoxia in someone who has a chest infection (e.g. PCP). Delirium should not be confused with dementia, and hallucinations, which may be caused by HIV encephalopathy or other infections, may also be drug induced. Some patients with early HIV encephalopathy appear to become very sensitive to psychotropic drugs. In these cases the introduction of new drugs must be undertaken with caution and in small doses. Some patients, especially those who are severely debilitated, quickly develop extra-pyramidal symptoms even at normal therapeutic doses of, for example, metoclopramide, prochlorperazine or haloperidol. It should be borne in mind that a possible cause of confusion could be drug interactions resulting from the polypharmacy that frequently has to be practised in treating people with AIDS.

HIV encephalopathy is frequently associated with vacuolar myelopathy where the patient may present with ataxia, incontinence and loss of power in the legs. Peripheral neuropathies are also very common; in some cases the symptoms remain minimal, in others they become extremely severe. A recent study (Scaravilli *et al.*, 1989) indicates that haemophiliacs with HIV disease may die before the development of the HIV related encephalopathy that is so common in others with advanced AIDS. They appear also to have a lower incidence of opportunistic infections affecting the CNS. This may be because they are at high risk of developing fatal intra-cranial haemorrhage before the onset or full development of HIV related neurological complications. It may also be that haemophiliacs are more likely to develop other diseases associated with blood transfusions such as hepatitis or cirrhosis of the liver.

Some studies (Portegies *et al.*, 1989) have indicated that Zidovudine may delay or prevent the onset of HIV encephalopathy in HIV positive individuals, and patients may wish to continue taking Zidovudine for as long as possible, even up until the time of death.

Kaposi's sarcoma (KS)

In the West 35 per cent of patients with AIDS are said to present with KS (Kaplan *et al.*, 1988). (KS is very much more common in homosexual patients than in others.) Patients who present with KS in a slowly progressive form on the skin generally have a better overall prognosis than patients who present with, for example, PCP or other opportunistic infections. However, when the KS is aggressive with pulmonary and other visceral involvement the prognosis is usually a matter of months at the most, although response to radiotherapy or chemotherapy may be good and prolong life by several months, or even a year or more. Obvious KS lesions on the face or other exposed parts of the body may

Table 5 HIV encephalopathy.

Early signs	Short-term memory loss intermittent confusion loss of concentration changes in personality and behaviour
Progression of encephalopathy	Diffuse neurological signs ataxia tremor limb weaknesses loss of co-ordination
Advanced encephalopathy	Total dementia Incontinence Grand mal attacks

be camouflaged with make-up. (Camouflage make-up and information may be obtained from, for example, the Red Cross, p.110.) Radiotherapy or chemotherapy may be used to improve appearance or to prevent deterioration, and to reduce swelling and discomfort. Chemotherapy may also reduce obstruction caused by oesophageal KS; chemotherapeutic agents such as Bleomycine, Vinblastine, or Vincristine are commonly used. Radiotherapy given to oral mucosa may cause breakdown and ulceration and should be used with caution.

When the patient's general condition indicates that he is rapidly approaching the terminal phase of his illness, and if swelling and discomfort from KS lesions is causing distress (e.g. facial or peri-orbital oedema) dexamethasone may be very effective in reducing swelling and discomfort, and in improving quality of life, albeit only for a short while.

Skin problems

Skin problems (see Table 6) are extremely common in AIDS. Kaposi's sarcoma (see above) affects the skin in a substantial number of people with AIDS. Viral skin infections, such as *Herpes simplex* and *Herpes zoster* (see pp. 54–55), are common and bacterial and fungal infections and eczema and psoriasis frequently occur. Recurring skin problems may be an early sign of HIV disease, but skin infections or other conditions are almost universal in advanced AIDS. Scabies should be borne in mind as a possible cause of any atypical rash (see below).

Dry skin is found in almost all patients with the advanced disease, but is particularly severe in those who have suffered a slowly progressive debilitating process with persistent diarrhoea and weight loss, may be as a result of malabsorption. The skin may be itchy and flaking, and therefore more vulnerable to secondary infection. Regular daily applications of moisturising cream and emollients applied to the skin or added to the bath may help to reduce itching and prevent secondary infection.

Seborrhoaeic dermatitis/eczema commonly appears as reddened, sometimes scaly or crusting patches between or around the eyebrows, nasolabial folds, and in the beard and scalp areas, particularly around the hairline. It is commonly associated with fungal or yeast infections, and is best treated with topical steroids and anti-fungal creams in combination (1 per cent Hydrocortisone to face, stronger steroids elsewhere). Scalp problems may be improved with the use of, for example, Selsun shampoo plus Betnovate scalp lotion or Synalar gel.

Folliculitis is a generalised pruritic eruption and may occur together with seborrhoaeic dermatitis. Folliculitis may have the same aetiology as seborrhoaeic dermatitis but it responds less well to treatment as the pruritus may be very severe. Anti-histamines may help to reduce the pruritis and applications of Eurax (Crotamiton) may be helpful. However, bear in mind the possibility of scabies.

Psoriasis may appear for the first time in a person with HIV disease. It should be treated with the usual preparations such as salicylic acid and coldtar, dithranol or strong topical steroids.

Molluscum contagiosum is caused by the pox virus. It is common on the face, but also appears elsewhere as small papules with a dimple in the centre, which may become unsightly, and also interfere with shaving in the male. They may be treated with careful application of phenol to the centre of the small papule using the tip of a sharpened orange stick. Repeated applications may be necessary – they may be painful and require local anaesthesia.

Tinea infections are extremely common and more aggressive than in the non-immunocompromised person. They may occur anywhere on the skin as ring-worm, between the toes or as an infection of the nails. In the terminally ill patient treatment of nail infections may not be appropriate as this requires long term treatment with Griseofulvin for many months. Itroconazole or fluconazole are alternatives and may be useful in any fungal skin infection which has become extensive. Antifungal creams, with or without steroids, should be applied regularly, 2 or 3 times a day for 2 to 3 weeks, to the affected areas.

Table 6 Common skin problems (other than KS and Herpes infections).

Condition	Cause	Treatment or comment
Dry skin	?Malnutrition due to persistent diarrhoea causing reduced tryglycerides	Control of diarrhoea, and nausea and vomiting; diet and appetite stimulants; emollients
Seborrhoaeic dermatitis	Often associated with fungal or yeast infections	Topical steroids and antifungal creams, Selsun shampoo, Betnovate scalp lotion
Folliculitis generalised (pruritic eruption)	Often associated with fungal or yeast infections	Anti-histamines, Eurax (Crotamiton) NB exclude scabies
Psoriasis	May appear for 1st time in HIV + ve person	Salicyclic acid, cold tar, Dithranol and strong topical steroids
Molluscum contagiosum	Pox virus	Phenol or Silver nitrate applications
Ringworm	Tinea	Fluconazole, Itraconazole, Griseofulvin and anti-fungal creams
Norwegian scabies or crusted scabies	Very high number of scabies mites in immuno-compromised individual; delay in diagnosis	Gamma benzene hexachloride applications × 3 initially followed by weekly applications for several months; possible need for strong topical steroids to reduce skin reactions

Scabies should be suspected when a patient presents with any atypical rash which has persisted, or when crusting or nodules are present. In an immunocompromised host scabies may develop into what is known as Norwegian or exaggerated, nodular or crusted scabies (Ran and Baird, 1986), which is very contagious because of the increased number of mites carried by each patient. In an immune competent host there are estimated to be under 50 female egg laying mites, whereas in Norwegian scabies the number of such mites may multiply to over 2 million per patient. The diagnosis may be delayed because the rash is

atypical or may mimic, for example, seborrhoaeic dermatitis. A diag
nosis should be made by looking for the mite in skin scrapings, o
scrapings obtained from under the nails. Treatment is more difficult i
an immunocompromised person as repeated applications of scabicid
may be necessary to eradicate the infection. In ordinary scabies 90 pe
cent of live mites are usually eradicated by one application of gamm
benzene hexachloride (Alexander, 1968); in Norwegian scabies it ma
be necessary to continue with repeated applications for up to 6 month;
Repeated applications may result in an irritant reaction for which it i
necessary to apply potent topical steroids as well as scabicide. A
mentioned above, Norwegian scabies is extremely contagious, not leas
because of the enormous number of mites shed in the scale into beddin
and furniture. Although the scabies mite is thought to have only a sho;
survival time outside the human body, in one unit caring for peopl
with AIDS, staff who had not been in contact with the infected patien
but had used the same furniture, or had stood by the bedside, becam
infected. Six members of staff and three other patients became infecte
before the source was identified and it took three months to eradicat
the infection from the unit. All patients, their partners or carers, an
the staff and their partners needed treatment with weekly application;
and all the furnishings, including carpets and easy chairs, had to b
treated. It is advisable that a dermatological opinion and supervisio
is sought early if Norwegian scabies is suspected in a setting wher
immunocompromised patients may be at risk.

Lymphomas

The most common type of lymphoma that occurs in AIDS is the hig
grade B cell lymphoma. The most common sites are in the CNS, bon
marrow, gastro-intestinal tract, liver, heart, lymph nodes and rectum
The lymphomas may occur in one site only or be disseminated. Th
prognosis is usually poor, less than one year, although good rates o
remission have been obtained with certain chemotherapeutic regimes.

Common symptoms and their control

Many of the symptoms encountered in advanced AIDS are those tha
would be encountered in any terminal care situation. Table 7 illustrate
some of the most commonly encountered symptoms in 100 consecutiv
admissions to a hospice unit. This section will not attempt to deal witl
every symptom in detail; nor will it seek to take the place of the excellen
books that are available dealing with therapeutics in terminal cancer o
other life threatening illnesses. Here the basic principles from which t
work will be outlined, giving some useful guidelines to those who ma
not be so familiar with this approach to care.

Many symptoms are directly related to a treatable cause, even in the terminal care situation. For example, *Herpes simplex* infections in the ano-rectal region cause severe pain on defaecation and tenesmus, often persisting long after defaecation. This pain is best treated with a course of acyclovir (400 mg–800 mg 5 times daily for 5 days). Analgesia may also be necessary until the acyclovir has taken effect. The pain caused by an anal fissure, may be soothed with lignocaine ointment or gel, but healing of the fissure will only be possible when the anus is no longer subjected to either the stretching associated with the passing of hard stools, or the masceration associated with frequent loose stools or watery diarrhoea. The anorexia and soreness of the mouth associated with *Candida* infections are best treated by controlling, as far as possible, the infection. Nausea and vomiting are frequently side effects of one or more of the many drugs that the patients are taking; where possible it may make a considerable difference to rationalise the number of drugs, perhaps reducing the dosages and the number of drugs being taken, or the times at which the drugs are being taken.

When it is not possible to eradicate the cause it is usually possible to control the symptoms.

Pain

A considerable variety of different pains are commonly encountered in AIDS, especially in advanced AIDS. It is important to identify the type, site, severity and persistence of the pain being described. Each pain should be clearly identified and, where possible, the patient should be asked to quantify the pain by placing it on, for example, a visual analogue scale from 0 to 10, where 0 equals no pain and 10 equals the worst pain ever felt. This scale can then be used to monitor the response to therapy.

Total body pain

Total body pain is a condition in which the patient is so overwhelmed and distressed by pain that it is felt to be 'everywhere', with no particular focus. Total body pain may be the patient's response to overwhelming emotional distress, but it should be taken extremely seriously and treated as an emergency. The physical effects are similar to those of someone 'going into shock'. Once the overwhelming nature of the pain or other distress compounding the pain has been dealt with effectively, it is then possible to identify and deal with the details. Assessment should be made thoroughly but as quickly as possible, and an appropriate analgesic such as diamorphine should be given at once, subcutaneously or intravenously where necessary, together with an antiemetic such as cyclizine, haloperidol or methotrimeprazine which also have a sedative effect.

Table 7   Common symptoms on admission (in order of frequency) N = 100

Symptom	No's (= %)	Comments
Pain		
Neuropathic pain	22	HIV related; tingling, numbness, hyperaesthesia
Pressure sore pain	12	Pain related to direct pressure and inflammation
Visceral pain (chest/abdo)	10	Associated with KS, lymphoma, constipation
'Total body pain'	9	Diffuse overwhelming distress
Headaches	8	Associated with raised ICP or encephalitis
Joint pains	7	HIV arthropathy, septic monarthriti × 1
Epigastric pain/retrosternal	7	Herpes, Candida, NSAI's, lymphoma
Myopathic	5	May be related to AZT
Ano-rectal	4	Herpes infection, anal fissure
Other common symptoms		
General debility/wt loss	61	Most patients in advanced AIDS
Anorexia	41	Often related to mood/depression
Confusion/dementia	29	Differential diagnosis important
Nausea/vomiting	21	Often drug induced or related to crypto sp. or other infection
Depression	20	Differentiate from grief/sadness
Skin problems		Other common problems include viral, tinea, and bacterial infection
Dry skin	19	
Seb. dermatitis	14	
Scabies	7	
Molluscum contagiosum	4	
Psoriasis	1	
Cough	19	Dry, persistent cough, dyspnoea, ?PCP
Diarrhoea	18	Some treatable causes: cryptosporidial difficult to control
Constipation	18	Opioid therapy – treat pro-actively
Dyspnoea	11	?PCP, ?anaemia, KS, TB or other infective cause
Paralysis	8	Associated with CVA, toxoplasmosis, PML or lymphoma, myelopathy
Patients admitted moribund	8	

Table 8   Analgesic staircase for persistent or recurrent pain (adapted from Swerdlow and Ventafridda (1987)).

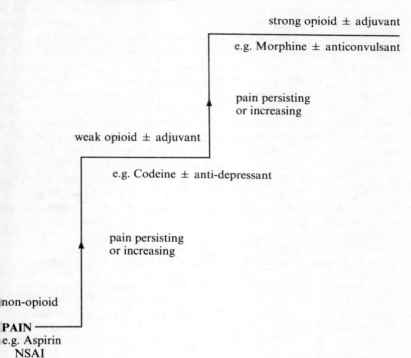

strong opioid ± adjuvant

e.g. Morphine ± anticonvulsant

pain persisting
or increasing

weak opioid ± adjuvant

e.g. Codeine ± anti-depressant

pain persisting
or increasing

non-opioid

PAIN
e.g. Aspirin
   NSAI

Persistent or recurring pain

'Persistent or recurring pain requires preventative therapy, i.e. analgesics should be given regularly and prophylactically. ''As required'' medication is irrational and inhumane in this situation.'
                                Twycross and Lack (1990)

'The aim is to titrate the dose of analgesic against the patient's pain, gradually increasing the dose until we obtain the maximum relief with the minimum interference'.
                                Swerdlow and Ventafridda (1987)

Morphine

The analgesic staircase (see Table 8) illustrates the process by which

pain may be controlled according to severity and response to analgesics
The response to therapeutic intervention should be monitored on a
frequent and regular basis (e.g. hourly or two hourly in severe pain
four hourly or daily as appropriate in less severe pain). Once the decision
has been taken to start morphine (or diamorphine), this should be given
orally every 4 hours (elixir, tablets or suppositories are also available)
It is usually recommended that 10 mg be given as a starting dose, but
this will depend on what analgesia the patient has already been taking
how effective it has been, and on the condition of the patient. In very
severely debilitated and emaciated patients smaller starting doses, such
as 2.5–5 mg, may be necessary as some patients appear to be particularly
sensitive and may develop unacceptable nausea and vomiting or drowsi-
ness. A regular anti-emetic, such as prochlorperazine or haloperidol
should be given with the morphine. However, the aim should be to
control the pain as quickly as possible, with as few side-effects as
possible. If the dose given has not controlled the pain by 80–90 per cent
the next increment up the table should be given. A chart for the
conversion between morphine and diamorphine is given in Table 9.

Table 9   Morphine and Diamorphine conversion chart; 4-hourly dose
equivalents.

Oral morphine (mg)	Injected diamorphine (mg)	Oral diamorphine (mg)
5	2·5	2·5
10	5	7·5
20	7·5	15
30	10	20
45	15	30
60	20	40
90	30	60
120	45	90

When pain control has been achieved and is being maintained on a
4 hourly regime it will be possible to change to sustained-release tablets
of morphine sulphate (MST continuous) – these are taken 12 hourly
and are therefore more convenient. The total dose taken over 24 hours
should be divided by 2 to obtain the 12 hourly dose. (MST tablets are
available as 10, 30, 60 and 100 mg.) (See also Table 9 for conversion to
diamorphine, oral and injected forms). It is usually possible to stop the
anti-emetic after a few days, unless other causes for nausea are present.

Adjuvants or co-analgesics

Some pains are resistant to opioids and respond better to combination with a co-analgesic or adjuvant drug. Table 10 shows the appropriate drug for the different types of pain. Rather than increasing the dose of opioid in the case of pain caused by the processes listed in Table 10, the addition of an appropriate co-analgesic drug may give much better pain control with fewer side-effects. For example, in the case of inflammatory or bone pains the addition of a non-steroidal anti-inflammatory agent may achieve better relief than morphine. To reduce the number of tablets taken, and the side-effects, the longer-acting forms should be used or those requiring only twice-daily dosages (e.g. sustained release indomethacin, naproxen, ketoprofen or diflunosal). It may also be useful to prescribe these drugs in suppository form, although not all patients will accept these. Naproxen has recently been used in a syringe driver with good results (Toscarni *et al.*, 1989).

Table 10 Adjuvants (co-analgesics) for some pain syndromes (adapted from Swerdlow and Ventafridda (1987)).

Type of pain	Adjuvant or co-analgesic indicated
Inflammatory or bone pain	Aspirin or NSAID
Raised intracranial pressure	Dexamethasone
Nerve destruction pain (deafferentation)	Antidepressants or/and anticonvulsants
Intermittent stabbing pain (neuralgic)	Anticonvulsants
Gastritis/PU Pain	Metoclopramide, Cimetidine, Ranitidine
Rectal/bladder spasm pain	Chlorpromazine
Muscle spasm pain	Diazepam, Baclofen

The anti-convulsants carbamazepine or sodium valproate are particularly useful for the control of neuropathic, neuralgic or deafferentation pains.

Dexamethasone is effective for the relief of headaches of raised intracranial pressure, for which opioids are not very effective. It is useful, also, for its powerful anti-inflammatory effect, and will improve appetite and induce a general sense of well being. Dexamethasone will also reduce the facial and orbital oedema that may be caused by KS lesions. There are dangers of long-term steroid use and of masking infective or inflammatory processes, but in the terminal care situation these may be out-weighed by the aim to improve quality of life.

Nausea and vomiting

Almost all patients with AIDS complain of nausea and vomiting at some stage, and for some it is extremely resistant to treatment. For many it is a transient problem but for some it is a continuing one, and contributes to anorexia and weight loss. It is important to diagnose the cause in order to prescribe the appropriate treatment. Table 11 illustrates the likely causes – drug induced nausea is the commonest, and that caused by, or associated with, cryptosporidial diarrhoea is probably the most difficult to control.

Table 11   The likely causes of nausea and vomiting (adapted from Swerdlow and Ventafridda (1987)).

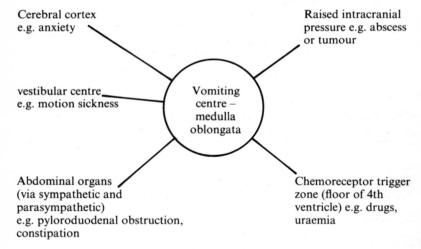

It may be possible to reduce or eliminate drug-induced nausea by rationalising the regime, simplifying it, or stopping certain drugs for a while. When other measures fail, adjusting the timing of drugs in relation to each other, or to meal-times, may be effective in reducing nausea and/or vomiting. Some drugs are available as suppositories and may be useful when the patient is vomiting, and/or objects to injections. The same rule applies to the treatment of nausea as to pain: it should be given regularly and not on a 'prn' basis, when it is persistent or recurrent in nature. Table 12 provides guidelines for the treatment of nausea and vomiting.

Intractable vomiting may be associated with, for example, cryptosporidial diarrhoea, or severe anxiety. A combination of anti-emetics, working at different levels may achieve better control than a single drug. In some cases it may be necessary to use a syringe driver to

Table 12   Treatment guidelines for nausea and vomiting. (Recommended drugs are examples only.)

Cause	Drug: dose recommended	Comment	Site of action of drugs (main)
METABOLIC e.g. drug induced e.g. uraemia carcinomatosis	Cyclizine 25–50 mg tds**	EP effects	Chemoreceptor trigger zone
	Prochlorperazine 5–25 mg	Sedative/EP effects	
	Chlorpromazine 25–50 mg*	Sedative/EP effects	
	Domperidone 10–30 mg tds+	No EP effects	
	Metoclopramide 10–20 mg tds*	EP effects (60 kg or less)	
	Methotrimeprazine 25–50 mg tds*	Very sedative	
	Haloperidol 0·5–5 mg bd*	EP effects/sedative	
ABDOMINAL e.g. constipation gastritis	Metoclopramide 10–20 mg tds*	Promotes peristalis and relaxes pylorus	Chemoreceptor trigger zone and local action
	Domperidone 10–30 mg tds+		
CORTICAL e.g. anxiety or psychological stimuli	Haloperidol 0.5–10 mg bd*	May cause EP effects at higher doses	Chemoreceptor trigger zone
	Prochlorperazine 5–25 mg tds*	Sedative	
	Chlorpromazine 25–50 mg tds*		
VESTIBULAR e.g. motion sickness	Cyclizine 25–50 mg tds	Drowsiness, dry mouth	Vomiting centre
	Cinnarizine		
	Dimenhydrinate 50–100 mg bd or tds		

+ does not cross blood-brain barrier
* may be used in syringe driver
** tendency to crystallise in syringe driver
EP = extrapyramidal

achieve good 24-hour control, and to enable a patient to eat and drink and to have some measure of quality. Once control has been achieved it may be possible to return to oral medication. Nabilone (1–2 mg PO) may be effective where other treatments fail, but may cause euphoria or other CNS effects (Green *et al.*, 1989).

Anorexia and weight loss

These very common problems may be treated with Megestrol acetate (40–80 mg bd–qds) which has been shown to increase weight as well as appetite (von Roenn *et al.*, 1988). Periactin (4 mg bd or tds) may also stimulate the appetite, as will prednisolone or dexamethasone. However, in very advanced disease it may not be possible to achieve significant results for long, if at all.

The use of a syringe driver

The use of the syringe driver in terminal care is a well established practice. It is very useful as a tool for delivering medication smoothly over 24 hours in order to
— to achieve symptom control when the patient is no longer able to take oral medication; and
— to control intractable vomiting and diarrhoea.
The medication is delivered sub-cutaneously through a 'butterfly' needle, the site of which should be changed whenever local skin reactions develop, which may be every few days, or once weekly. In those for whom skin reaction is a problem the addition of 1500 i.u. of hyalase to the syringe driver may reduce the reaction and prolong the time available at a particular site.

Drugs which have been found to be effective when using syringe drivers in the terminal care of patients with AIDS are given below.

Diamorphine More soluble than morphine, and used to control pain, diarrhoea and dyspnoea.

Hyoscine For reducing secretions in pneumonia or chest infections; also may help to control diarrhoea, and to reduce peristalsis in intestinal obstructions or severe colicky pain.

Methotrimeprazine Very effective anti-emetic, and sedative in terminal restlessness.

Cyclizine Effective, but has a tendency to crystallise in the needle or 'butterfly' tube unless well diluted.

Metoclopramide Effective and will mix with other commonly used drugs in the syringe driver.

Haloperidol Useful in anxious, agitated or psychotic patients, as well as to control drug induced emesis; will also mix with other drugs.

Chlorpromazine May be used for its sedative and anti-emetic properties.

Midazolam (Ainsbury and Dunfy, 1989). Useful for agitation and restlessness, or as an anti-convulsant in those who require one. Diazepam pr may also be used (4–8 hourly) to achieve similar control and will cause muscle relaxation (more effectively than midazolam) in someone with increased muscle tone, or in neck retraction.

Phenobarbitone May be used in a syringe driver but should not be mixed with other drugs.

The reader is referred to the reading list on p. 107 for further information about detailed symptom-control matters. In the care of someone with AIDS, as in any terminal care situation, it is the meticulous attention to detail, the degree of good communication between all concerned, and the teamwork, with compassion and understanding, which will make the ultimate difference to the quality of living and the dying, and the memories with which the patient's loved ones have to live in the years to follow.

Table 13 provides a summary of drugs which are used for the treatment of common problems associated with AIDS and HIV infection.

Psychiatric Problems

These are too complex to be detailed here. Suffice it to say that they are common, and close liaison must be set up and maintained with psychiatric services and psychologists with an understanding of HIV related issues. A basic understanding of the use of psychotropic drugs is essential, and differentiation between psychiatric and organic disease is often difficult.

Table 13 Drugs used for the treatment of common problems associated with AIDS and HIV infection.

Drug	Used for	Doses	Side effects	Interactions
Zidovudine (Retrovir, AZT)	ARC or AIDS Inhibits Replication of HIV virus	(1) 200 mg 4 hrly (2) 3·5 mg/kg 4 hrly (3) Now often used qds, tds or bd regime. Reduced dose if signs of toxicity	Haematological – anaemia Neutropenia, leucopenia, thrombocytopenia, Nausea, vomiting, anorexia, abdominal pain, headaches, rashes and pruritus. Fever, myalgia, insomnia	Increased risk of toxicity with other nephrotoxic and myelosuppressive drugs Probencid increases plasma levels. Avoid chronic paracetamol use – increases toxicity Caution with drugs that have hepatic glucuronidation
Co-Trimoxazole (Septrin)	Acute PCP	60 mg/kg IV bd or 480 mg × 8 bd PO for 14–21 days	Nausea, vomiting, fever, rash, leucopenia, thrombocytopenia, abnormal LFTs	Possible potentiation of Hypoglycaemics, Phenytoin, Warfarin and Methotrexate
	Prophyllaxis	960 mg bd PO		
Pentamidine	Acute PCP	IV 4 mg/kg/day over at least one hour for 14 days	Hypotension (can be severe) Hypo or hyperglycaemia, phlebitis, rash, nausea, vomiting, nephrotoxicity	Nephrotoxicity and hypocalcaemia more likely with Foscarnet
		Nebulised: 600 mg in 6 ml sterile water for 14 days	Bronchospasm (pre-treatment with β2 agonist may reduce this)	
	Prophyllaxis	Nebulised: 300 mg in 3 ml sterile water every fortnight	As above	

Table 13 continued

Drug	Used for	Doses	Side effects	Interactions
Foscarnet	CMV Infections	Depends on creatinine clearance	Nephrotoxicity Anaemia Hypo/hypercalcaemia Phlebitis Headaches	Nephrotoxicity and hypocalcaemia, more likely if concurrent Pentamidine is given
Acyclovir (Zovirax)	Acute *Herpes simplex* and zoster infections	400–800 mg PO Five times a day for 5–7 days (also IV). Topical cream	Rashes. GI disturbances Abnormal LFTs Renal impairment Neurological reactions	Probenecid increases plasma levels
	Prophyllaxis	200–400 mg bd–qds		
Ketoconazole (Nizoral)	Acute Candidiasis Various mycoses	200 mg bd with food	Rashes, pruritis, GI disturbances, gynaecomastia Few reports of fatal liver damage	Reduced absorption with high pH (Antacids, H_2 antagonists) Rifampicin increases metabolism. Enhanced anti-coagulation with Warfarin and Nicoumalone. Phenyotoin enhanced and plasma Ketoconazole concentration reduced
	Prophyllaxis	200 mg od with food		

Table 13 continued

Drug	Used for	Doses	Side effects	Interactions
Dapsone	Acute PCP (combined with Trimethoprim) Prophyllaxis – PCP	100 mg PO/day	Nausea, vomiting, anaemia (NB G6PD-deficiency) Methaemoglobinaemia, neuropathy, headache, agranulocytosis, hepatitis	Probenicid slows urinary excretion. Nitrates and Nitrofurantoin may increase the risk of haemolysis in G6PD deficiency
Fansidar Pyrimethamine 25 mg Sulfadoxine 500 mg	PCP Prophyllaxis Toxoplasmosis	1 tablet weekly 2 Tablets bd for 3 weeks. 1 Tablet od maintenance for life	Rash. Stevens-Johnson Syndrome, bone marrow, depression, neutropenia	Folate antagonists may increase risk of haematological side effects. Folinic acid may be preventative
Gancyclovir (DHPG)	CMV infections Acute Maintenance	IV 5 mg/kg bd for 10–20 days IV 5 mg/kg od five days a week	Bone marrow depression, neutropenia and thrombocytopenia, nausea and vomiting. Phlebitis, eosinophilia, reversible LFT abnormalities and testicular atrophy	Other myelosuppressive drugs Smaller doses are being tried

Table 13 continued

Drug	Used for	Doses	Side effects	Interactions
Itraconazole (Sporanox)	Acute Candidiasis Various Mycoses	200 mg od	Nausea, abdominal pain, dyspepsia and headaches	Antacids reduce absorption. Rifampicin accelerates metabolism. H$_2$ antagonists reduce absorption
	Prophyllaxis	100 mg od		
Fluconazole (Diflucan)	Acute Candidiasis Various Mycoses	Up to 400 mg per day in divided doses	Nausea, abdominal discomfort, headache. Occasionally abnormal LFTs	Enhanced effect of Phenytoin. Nicoumalone and Warfarin enhanced
	Prophyllaxis	50 mg od		
Amphotericin Lozenges (Funglin)	Oropharyngeal Candidiasis	Up to 8 lozenges per day	Few except with IV administration	Increased risk of nephrotoxicity with aminoglycosides
Nystatin Suspension/Pastilles	Oral Candida	1–5 mls qds One pastille qds	Nausea and vomiting in high doses	

References

Ainsbury, B. D. W. and Dunfy, K. P. (1989). The use of sub cutaneous Midazolam in the home care setting. *Palliative Medicine*, **3**, 299–301.

Alexander, S. (1968). Clinical trial of a scabicide. *Medical World*, **106(7)**, 20–4.

Gabuzda, D. H. and Hirsch, M. S. (1987). Neurological manifestations of infection with HIV. *Annals of International Medicine*, **107**, 383–9.

Green, S. T., Nathwarn, D., Goldberry, D. J. (1989). Nabilone as effective therapy for intractable nausea and vomiting in AIDS (Letter). *British Journal of Clinical Pharmacology*, **28(4)**, 494–5.

Kaplan, L. B. *et al.* (1988). Kaposi's sarcoma involving the lung in patients with the acquired immuno-deficiency syndrome. *Journal of Acquired Immuno-Deficiency Syndromes*, **1**, 23–30.

Lantos, P. L., McLaughlin, J. E., Scholtz, C. L. *et al.* (1989). Neuropathology of the brain in HIV infection. *Lancet*, **1(8633)**, 309.

Meunier-Carpentier, F. (1984). Chemoprophylaxis of fungal infection. *American Journal of Medicine*, **76**, 652–6.

Mulvenna, P. and Moss, V. A. (1992). AIDS-related diarrhoea: a rational approach to symptomatic treatment. (letter.) *Palliative Medicine* **6**, 260–61.

O'Neill, W. M. (1992). AIDS related diarrhoea: a rational approach to symptomatic treatment. *Palliative Medicine* **6**, 61–4.

Portegies, P., De Gans, J. Lange, J. M. A. *et al.* (1989). Declining instance of AIDS dementia complex after introduction of Zidovudine treatment. *British Medical Journal*, **299(6703)**, 819–21.

Ran, R. C. and Baird, I. M. (1986). Crusted scabies in HIV infection. *Journal of American Academy of Dermatology*, **15**, 1050–9.

Scaravilli, F., Esiri, M. M., Millard, P. R. (1989). Neuropathology of HIV infection in haemophiliacs. Comparative necropsy study. *British Medical Journal*, **299(6711)**, 1312.

Swerdlow, M. and Ventafridda, V. (Eds) (1987). *Cancer Pain*. MTP Press Ltd, Lancaster, UK.

Toscarni, F., Barosi, K., Scazzini, M. (1989). Sodium naproxen: Continuous sub cutaneous infusion in neoplastic pain control. *Palliative Medicine*, **3**, 207–11.

Twycross, R. and Lack, S. (1990). *Therapeutics in Cancer Care*, second edition. Churchill Livingstone, Edinburgh.

von Roenn, J. H. *et al.* (1988). Megestrol acetate for treatment of cachexia associated with human immuno-deficiency virus infection. *Annals of Internal Medicine*, **109**, 840–1.

Youle, M., Farthing, C., Clarbour, J. and Wade, P. (1988). *AIDS: Therapeutics in HIV Disease*. Churchill Livingstone, Edinburgh.

7 Counselling

What is counselling in the setting of terminal care for people with AIDS? In this situation counselling is the facilitation of a personal understanding of, adjustment to, and acceptance of the disease and its effect upon their lives, by the patients, the people important to them, and those caring for them. It is not the intention in this chapter to discuss how to counsel, but rather to highlight the particular needs and problems when caring for a person who is terminally ill with AIDS. Whilst most of the issues involved will be issues confronting any person with a life threatening illness, there are differences which must be recognised and not underestimated. Despite attempts to educate and enlighten at national and local levels there still exists much fear and ignorance about AIDS and its transmission, even among health care professionals. This affects and often isolates patients and their families. Another difference was described very succinctly by Dr David Miller.

In the West AIDS is associated with traditionally marginalised and oppressed social groups, subject to prejudice and cultural and legal oppression. Often our patients, as members of society, will have internalised many of those prejudices and those negative social attitudes about them, and so a diagnosis of AIDS will act as a catalyst for the expression of that internalised prejudice. It will result in a heightened potential for self destruction, whether it be in the form of an active response such as suicide, or a more passive response, such as self destructive guilt, self hate or self pity.'

David Miller, personal communication

People with AIDS and their families live in constant uncertainty as to how and when the virus will affect them next and whether they will be able to cope. They also live with the perceived certainty that a diagnosis of AIDS equals death. Uncertainty may prove very difficult for many patients to live with, living with HIV antibody positive status, fearing every cough and cold and wondering when and if AIDS will be diagnosed. It may be a relief when the person knows that they have AIDS rather than living with uncertainty.

Counselling should be available at all stages of this illness, from pre-screening counselling to bereavement support and counselling. The input to psychological and emotional care and support of people with AIDS and their families is often enormous, and clearly cannot always be given by fully qualified counsellors or psychologists. Staff of other disciplines within the team will often be engaged in activities relating to counselling, and it is important that opportunities are given to these staff to increase their knowledge and skills related to listening and counselling. It is essential, however, that team members, even those skilled at counselling, know when to refer patients on to the counsellor or psychologist, who can concentrate entirely on the psychological and emotional needs of the patients and those close to them.

The emotional needs of these terminally ill patients must be responded to wherever they are being cared for. Whilst in a few hospitals and community services, statutory service provision is made to help meet these needs, in others very little help is available. If patients are being cared for at home most of their help will come from the primary care team or from voluntary organisations offering support and counselling help. In some areas specialised home care teams are available and, as part of their remit, they offer emotional support and help.

In order to identify the feelings people with AIDS may commonly deal with, consider the factors that will create and/or influence those feelings:

— the shock of facing their mortality
— despair and hopelessness relating to the absence of a cure
— anxiety about the implications for family and friends
— grief relating to present and anticipated losses
— fear of the mode of dying
— anger at having been given infected blood or blood products and/or at being the unlucky one, being caught out
— guilt; have I infected others?
— loss of self esteem and feelings of uselessness
— social isolation; real or perceived.

Whatever their coping mechanisms people with AIDS are likely to be experiencing much grief. The Oxford English dictionary describes grief as 'deep sadness'. In these circumstances the deep sadness of a person with AIDS is very understandable.

Peter is a young boy with haemophilia who now has AIDS. He is familiar with hospitals, having had repeated hospital admissions and is familiar with pain and disability. He has been excluded from certain activities and sports all of his life and, after repeated haemorrhages into his joints, he can now only walk with difficulty. Peter and his family have lived, and coped quite well, with fear, uncertainty and losses up to now. Now at 16 years of age he is dying. He has AIDS and the fears, social isolation and pain, both physical and emotional, associated with AIDS are touching him and his family. Peter and his parents are only able to share the diagnosis with a few key people, mainly those involved with his health and education. His parents have had to give him a lot of their time and feel guilty about his brother James. His mother describes the deep sadness she feels that, at only 19 years of age, James left home because of his own increasing isolation and pain as Peter became more ill.

Stress, grief and separation are putting pressure on the marriage. The parents describe it as 'rocky'.

Tracey has AIDS. She is now 19 years old but looks much older. Tracey used to live in squalor with her mother and two older brothers in a large council estate in Edinburgh.

When she was twelve, in common with most of her school friends on the estate, she became involved in solvent abuse; 'We all did it, it was better than nothing, and there was nothing to do.' From there she went on to experiment with drugs and finally, at sixteen, she became addicted to heroin and shared 'works' with her friends. In order to finance her drug habit she became a prostitute, and stole goods and money from wherever she could, including her home.

Tracey's relationship with her mother became more and more impossible as her life-style became more chaotic and eventually, as she put it, 'Mum chucked me out'.

Tracey came to London when she was seventeen: with no money and no friends. She was given a home by a man who promised her food, and money to finance her drugs which she earned by giving her 'services' to him and to his clients. When Tracey became ill and was found to have AIDS she was again 'chucked out' and became homeless. After treatment in hospital Tracey registered at a drug dependency unit and is now taking reducing doses of Methadone. She is self caring, but suffers from chronic tiredness and diarrhoea, and is living on her own in bed and breakfast accommodation. Tracey misses her mother and her friends but feels that she cannot go back now that she has AIDS.

Chris is 25 years old. He is a gay man and he has AIDS. For as long as he can remember he has felt different from other boys but he kept these feelings to himself and worried a lot. At 16 years of age he discussed these feelings with the family doctor who told him not to worry, he would 'grow out of it'.

Chris's parents had separated when he was fourteen and he had lived with his mother who was a teacher, and a strict Roman Catholic. He wanted so much to be 'normal', but finally decided he must accept himself as he was. Chris felt very sad about this as he loved children and wanted to be married and have a family, and now felt his homosexuality would deny him this. At the age of 20 Chris decided to talk with his mother about his situation. Her response was to cry, to hurl abuse at him and to distance herself from him. There had been a lot of press coverage about AIDS and it worried her. She decided that, despite the fact that he told her that he did not have a 'relationship' with anyone, he must have his own cutlery, crockery and towels etc. Every time he took a bath or went to the toilet his mother would clean the area with neat bleach.

Chris was a gentle, sensitive boy and it grieved him deeply that the one person he loved most in the world should reject him. He felt that God had rejected him too. Eventually his mother asked him to leave the home and Chris went to live with his father and his father's new wife. They allowed him to stay, but made him feel uncomfortable with their unkind comments and eventually, having got a good job, Chris rented a flat of his own. Rejected by society and by his own family he sought relationships that would be meaningful and fulfilling. After a series of disastrous relationships Chris met Martin who was also 21 years of age. They set up home together. The following 18 months were the happiest Chris had known. He was loved and cared for and about and felt secure in that love. Suddenly Chris became ill – he had diarrhoea and lost a lot of weight. He had been feeling tired lately and seemed to have no energy. Chris then got pneumonia and his worst fears were realised. He had AIDS; had he infected Martin? Martin was devastated. Here they were on the brink of life together with so much promise and it was all coming to an end. Chris wrote to his mother, but the letter was returned unopened.

Looking at these scenarios should enable the carer to see the other issues that many people with AIDS will need to work through including

— child abuse
— separation
— rejection
— isolation
— disability
— drug and alcohol abuse
— loss.

The role of the counsellor

Whilst it is important that counselling should be available, not all patients will need, or wish, to use the service, and although the patient or client may have many problems with which to deal, they cannot all be dealt with at once. The patient will indicate where he wants to start by introducing issues that he is ready to face and the counsellor must proceed only at this pace. Patients need time to help them face their losses and start the grieving process. Sigmund Freud talked about grief work – the idea of grief as a job of work which needs to be done if a person is to come through and get on with his or her life. Dr Colin Murray Parkes (personal communication) put it another way: 'It is a process of re-learning, it's a way of facing and coping with the new world which we are now entering, however much we may be reluctant to enter that world'. The role of the counsellor in this context, therefore, is to facilitate that re-learning and to help patients and their loved ones through the process of facing and coping with grief and loss.

Coping mechanisms may commonly be manifested in denial and anger. People with AIDS may move in and out of denial, only sometimes feeling able to attempt to face reality. Anger presents in many ways and

an affect all the patients' relationships. He may be looking for someone
r something to blame and anyone will do. Anger can be disruptive
nd cause much pain and hurt to the people who matter most to the
atient. If a patient is able to see that, in this situation, anger is
nderstandable and is part of grieving, he will be better able to deal with
. Most patients appreciate having someone who wants to listen to
em, someone who is interested in what they have to say, someone
ho has the time. Some, however, may find talking very difficult, or be
epressed and/or withdrawn. For these people it is important just to
e there', keeping the care on offer and ensuring that they have access
the carer. Patients who have experienced social and emotional depri-
ation and have a poor self image may need more help in coping with
eir grief. Counsellors who anticipate the problems that they are going
meet, and the situations they are likely to confront, are likely to be
etter prepared when they do meet these situations. The person who is
erminally ill with AIDS will also be better able to cope when he has
ad opportunities to discuss with a counsellor the anticipated problems
r fears.

The counsellor should have considerable input to the care of those who
re close to the patient. Family therapy, involving several members of
he same family, is often needed. Lack of understanding and intolerance,
ong standing conflicts and separations and collusion between family
nembers will often prevent the family from supporting the patient and
ach other. The complexity of relationships amongst the patients may
nean that those who are close to the patient will have many emotional
roblems. Particular problems which with the counsellor may be faced
nclude the following.

— Male patients may have an ex-wife, young children, parents, a
  partner and an ex-partner, all of whom he may care about, and
  the counsellor may need to be involved with all of these people.

— Parents, who may be elderly and/or disabled themselves, sometimes
  for the first time facing the fact that their son is gay, are now also
  confronted with the fact that he is dying.

— Parents, still young themselves, and brothers and sisters are re-
  united after several years with their daughter/son or sister/brother
  who is now terminally ill.

— Partners of patients, who may themselves be HIV antibody
  positive, watching the effect of the disease on the one they love.
  They have often had other close friends who have died and may
  still be grieving for them. Patients may have lived with their partner
  for many years and have had little contact with their family. At
  this time patients will often be re-united with their families, however
  the partner may be rejected by the family. The counsellor should
  be in a position to help the individuals concerned to deal with their

conflict and bring harmony to the situation, although this is n
always possible, usually because the parents/siblings are unwillin
or unable to accept the partner. It is important to ensure that th
wishes of the patient are respected and, if in hospital or a hospic
to arrange for separate visiting times for the partner and the famil
if necessary.

— Families of people with AIDS are seldom able to talk freely abou
their son's/daughter's illness and/or death in their own home tow
hence may become isolated from friends and their support.

— Women with children who are HIV positive may be overwhelme
by a sense of personal guilt, 'I have infected my own child,' or b
anger directed at the partner who infected them both.

— As it is very difficult to identify the terminal stage of AIDS patien
and their families may need counselling to help adjust to situation
where apparent imminent death gives place to recovery.

Bereavement support and follow up

Whenever possible bereavement support should begin before the patien
dies. As stated earlier, if people are prepared for events they are muc
more likely to be able to cope with them. The families and friends o
many people with AIDS have very little social support available. Ga
organisations have set-up support networks for gay men who are HIV
antibody positive; this work has developed and now also offers suppor
to heterosexual men and women. The value of group support canno
be underestimated. Organisations offering help include the following:
— Cruse
— Positive Partners
— BAHN (Black AIDS and HIV Network)
— Mainliners
— Body Positive
— Positively Women
— Terrence Higgins Trust
— London Lighthouse
— Mildmay Mission Hospital (see Appendix 1).
Memorial services and social evenings for relatives and friends of peopl
who have died, and support groups for partners can assist in thi
bereavement process. Trained bereavement support volunteers, visiting
people at home and referring back to counsellors if further in-put i
needed, may also be of value.

Identifying the grief and loss people with AIDS and those close to
them may experience can be a painful process in itself. The reader could
be forgiven for thinking that being involved in the terminal care o
people with AIDS is a thoroughly unhappy and depressing arena o

are to be in – it is not. People with AIDS often have amazing courage and determination. They are fighters – fighting for life. They do not sit round with counsellors 'coming to terms' with things; instead they are concerned with living. They are caring for, and about, those they love, caring about each other, and giving the carer the privilege of sharing in their lives.

> A patient had just finished drawing a rainbow.
>   'There's one thing missing, though,' he said.
>   'And what's that?' asked the counsellor who was visiting him.
>   'A crock of gold.'
>   'What would you do with the crock of gold?'
>   'I'd spend it.'
>   'And what would you spend it on?'
>   'Life.'

Acknowledgements

Acknowledgement is made to the lectures on 'Bereavement and loss' given by Dr Colin Murray Parkes; and that on 'Counselling' given by Dr David Miller at the conference 'Terminal care for AIDS patients: An Holistic Approach' held in January 1988 at the Mildmay Mission Hospital.

8   Spiritual and pastoral care

'Even though I walk through the valley of the shadow of death, I will
fear no evil, for you are with me....'

Psalm 23

In providing for the needs of the whole person the importance of
spiritual and pastoral needs must be recognised. Even the person who
has no faith in a God, and is quite content in his or her atheism, has a
world view, a system of beliefs about the world, social systems, and his
or her place in them. A person's world view and belief system has a
profound effect on the way in which he or she faces issues of physical
illness, death and dying. Facing death can also challenge deeply and
long-held beliefs as nothing else can. It is then of the greatest importance
that there are people available to share that challenge, to listen while
he or she struggles with the often unanswerable questions of life, such
as 'Why me?' The question: 'If there is a loving God why does he allow
me, his child, to suffer like this?' may be asked. Usually, the answer can
only be 'I don't know'. Christians may share the conviction that God
suffers with the patient and that He wants to be there to help carry the
pain, seeing God's answers in the Cross and the Resurrection, giving
hope. The words, however, will only become reality through the carers
actions, their presence, acceptance and sharing of the pain. This is
where faith without works is indeed dead, and will mean nothing to the
person who is suffering unless it is backed up by practical action.

The person with AIDS may be facing particular spiritual conflicts
and emotional pain as a result of condemnation and rejection throughout their lives. This condemnation and rejection may have been expressed by the churches or the religious communities in which they have
grown up. Society's fear of AIDS has meant that people with AIDS are
often extremely isolated. This is true for all who are affected by AIDS.
The parent whose child is dying with AIDS may, with good reason,
fear the results of telling their neighbours or even their church fellowship
or friends what the real problem is. Elderly parents have been known
to tell their neighbours and friends that their son was dying from cancer
because this would at least ensure them sympathy. The single mother
with AIDS who has one or two children, struggles alone for fear of her
children being taken into care and the reaction of neighbours should it
become known that she has AIDS and that her children may be HIV
positive. Sadly, some Christians have only compounded the sense of

solation by their attitude and their pre-occupation with judgement and theological discussion about innocence and guilt, right and wrong. The person with AIDS, therefore, is particularly vulnerable and sensitive, and may be afraid to speak or acknowledge spiritual needs.

As well as the fear that many people have of acknowledging and talking about spiritual issues, many will also have a deep sense of anger; anger at their God, anger at their particular religious community, represented by, for example, ministers of religion or chaplains. This anger may have to be expressed and accepted before any useful work can begin.

It is important that the multiprofessional team acknowledges that a person who is facing death has spiritual issues that need to be dealt with, and to make provision for these needs to be met. The person who is dying will choose with whom he speaks about such matters; it may be the home-help, it may be the nurse or the doctor. It will certainly not be with anyone from whom he fears ridicule or condemnation and he may well be afraid of speaking with a chaplain or recognised minister of religion. It is therefore important that the spiritual counsellors or ministers of religion to whom a person may be referred are known to be sympathetic and understanding of the issues involved.

The hospice movement has done much to increase our understanding of the spiritual needs of people facing death. Several excellent books which deal with these issues in general, or in particular, are available (see Further reading) and provide a deeper coverage of the subject than is possible in this chapter. This chapter considers the *practice of spiritual and pastoral care* for someone who is living with AIDS and has to face issues of death and dying.

The carer must learn not to make assumptions or to use jargon.

A young woman had had little apparent experience of security, love or beauty. She said that she did not believe in God, but expressed fear of death, of hell and the afterlife. The concept of a loving father meant nothing to her; in her experience the word 'father' was associated with abuse and neglect. It took time and patience to build up trust before any of these issues could be dealt with and then they could only be dealt with on a very simple basis. Theological discussion would have lost her completely. What she needed and wanted was love expressed in practical care, someone to sit and hold her hand in the dark when she was afraid at night to go to sleep, to read Psalm 23 to her when she wanted it, at her request to pray simply for God's acceptance of her, and to prove it by our continuing acceptance of her. This involved the whole team, and the people she chose particularly to talk with were those older members of the team who could represent to her a mother figure. The chaplain, too, played an important role in pastoral care and in planning with her her funeral and then taking it from Mildmay. She wanted Psalm 23 to be read at her funeral, and for all of us who were able to attend it left an indelible memory.

The role of the Minister of Religion in the multiprofessional team

For ease of reference the minister of religion or spiritual counsellor will be referred to as the Chaplain. In a hospice the Chaplain may be residential and a full member of the multiprofessional team, attending team meetings and being available to patients, their families and to staff on a regular and daily basis. Alternatively, hospices and hospitals may work with the local clergy and visiting chaplains, with ministers of religion from a variety of denominations or religions on call when required. In the community it is useful for the primary care teams to build up good links and liaison with the local clergy with whom they can work and to whom they can refer people when appropriate. However, as mentioned previously, it is essential that the attitudes and understanding of the Chaplains or the Clergy likely to be involved are fully understood.

The role of the Chaplain includes providing for the religious needs (sacramental, ceremonial and ritual) that people have at this time, arranging funeral services, providing support and pastoral care for the patients, their families, partners and friends, liaising with other chaplains, ministers of religion and spiritual counsellors where appropriate, and last but not least, in just being there and available as a friend and supporter when needed and wanted.

Sacraments and rituals

Sacraments and rituals vary from religion to religion and from denomination to denomination, and may assume a greater meaning than ever before to someone who is living with AIDS and facing issues of death and dying. They may reinforce a sense of security and belonging and provide the means for expressing deeply felt beliefs without the need for discussion or exploration; they may serve, also, as a trigger to further discussion and exploration. Within the Christian tradition there may be the need for communion, confession and absolution administered by a priest; for some patients the services of Baptism and Confirmation will provide vehicles for establishing or re-establishing their sense of commitment to a system of beliefs; regular and special services may help and uplift; and for some anointing with oil and prayer for healing may be very important. Most religions have their own rituals and the chaplain may be needed to coordinate or facilitate these, bringing in the appropriate person to administer them at the patient's request. In many religions the last rites are of utmost importance and these must be respected by the people involved in providing care at this time.

Funeral services

As there may be some clergy and funeral directors who are unwilling to be involved in the funeral of someone who has died of AIDS, it is important to establish links early, discussing all issues at length and in depth. The funeral service should be conducted sensitively and with full understanding of the families/partners feelings and needs, including the full recognition of the partner's place in the person's life regardless of the legal status or general acceptance of that partnership. For many people living with AIDS, an important part of their positive approach is to think through and plan their funeral service, and the chaplain has an important role in facilitating this. Not all patients can do this however, and it is important for the families and partners to be able to turn to the chaplain knowing that he or she is familiar with their situations. Some patients may not wish to have a religious service. Some may want a celebration of their life instead of a funeral service and this may be a very moving and positive expression of their personality. There are now organisations that advise and help with secular funerals (see Appendix 1). Any rituals or ceremonies that are important to the person and those surrounding him should be given recognition through provision of time and space for these to take place.

Pastoral counselling and support

Pastoral counselling should be available to the person with AIDS, his family, partner and friends and others who may be important to him, and may provide a vehicle by which deeper spiritual care can be given. Pastoral counselling involves listening, sometimes counselling, often just being there and available. Sometimes it will take the form of very practical support such as providing company, taking someone for a drive, playing a game of scrabble or chess. These activities may all form part of the 'bridge of friendship' over which deeper communication can take place and through which trust and understanding can be developed. It is possible to 'hide' behind the ceremonies or rituals, so as to avoid dealing with deeper spiritual or pastoral issues. Collusion between the chaplain, the patient and those close to him may enable the chaplain, as well as the patient, to avoid dealing with painful or difficult subjects. Ainsworth-Smith and Speck (1982), in their book *Letting go*, identify four basic pastoral functions.

Reconciliation　To facilitate a sense of reconciliation between the person and God, between him and those with whom he is in relationship, and within himself, with assurance of forgiveness.

Sustaining　To support through personal presence and understanding, and through the administration of the sacraments, where appropriate.

Guidance   To explain and/or guide the person through his exploration of belief and faith.

Growth   To promote growth in maturity and wholeness.

Ainsworth-Smith and Speck feel that when time is short, as with someone who is facing imminent death, the focus should be on reconciliation and assurance. Pastoral support and counselling will facilitate this and may do much to promote the growth of faith and wholeness.

The attributes and needs of the pastoral carer

In providing spiritual care for terminally ill people with AIDS, chaplains, parish priests and/or ministers of religion should have sensitivity and wisdom, and have dealt, or be dealing, with such issues as sexuality, issues of death and dying, of loss and disability. They should have faced issues of sexuality within themselves and their own mortality. They should have an understanding and appreciation of their own ministry and pastoral identity, as well as of other religions, world views and belief systems. Pastoral carers should be aware of their own body language which may express their feelings on such subjects as homosexuality, guilt and innocence. Chaplains should understand and accept the anger, rejection and suspicion that they will often meet in those who feel themselves to have been rejected and condemned by the Church or by their own religious communities, and often by their own families. Providers of pastoral care should be sincerely non-judgemental and accepting in their attitudes, and realise that the terminal care setting is not the arena for debates or statements on moral issues, but rather for comfort and strong reassurance.

Hospice and Hospital Chaplains, in particular, will need to have personal support as they themselves are facing conflict and questions which often arouse deep emotions. They may find their own strongly held beliefs challenged and their own identity threatened. They also will be facing multiple loss and bereavement having to conduct frequent funeral services for people who may have become friends. It is, therefore, important that the Chaplain involved in this arena of care has a good personal support network and the support and understanding of the multiprofessional team.

The needs of staff and carers

Staff and carers involved in terminal care for people with AIDS will also be facing the same issues and challenges and may need pastoral support. They may need someone with whom they can discuss spiritual, ethical and moral issues. They may need someone to cry with and to pray with.

Thus the chaplain or minister of religion involved in the terminal care of someone with AIDS has a deeply challenging and vital role to play in the whole care of the person and all those who surround him.

Reference

Ainsworth-Smith, I. and Speck, P. (1982). *Letting go*. Society for the Promotion of Christian Knowledge, London.

9 Practical issues related to death and dying

Much of the trauma and grief, and sometimes anger, that people feel at the time of bereavement, and which may be remembered vividly, often forever, is related to the practical issues surrounding death. It is important for all those involved in planning and setting up services for people with AIDS to have thought through, planned for and made policies relating to a number of practical issues. Some of these have been mentioned in other chapters but will be dealt with more fully here. Whilst many people with AIDS come from comfortable home situations and are surrounded by family and friends some will be homeless, some will have no friends or family nearby, or with whom they have any contact, some will be living in squalid surroundings, and some may be single parents struggling to cope on their own with children who are perhaps also HIV positive or have AIDS. Wherever terminal care is being given, whether it be in a hospital, in a hospice or in the home, the following matters need to have been thought about and planned for.

In preparation

Sorting out wills and other legal matters may weigh very heavily on someone who is facing their own imminent death. A member of the multiprofessional team, perhaps the social worker or counsellor, should ensure that there are appropriate forms available for those who wish to prepare their will, or to give power of attorney to a next of kin or other person of their choice. People with AIDS may require access to legal advice, but it is important to ensure that the solicitors involved are aware of and sympathetic about the issues related to AIDS. Serious family conflicts and traumas can be avoided if these matters are dealt with sensitively and properly by people who have experience in helping those who are affected by AIDS. Families may contest a will if property or substantial sums of money have been left to a partner or a charity of whom the family do not approve. Those involved in a patient's care, particularly if working for a charity or organisation which may have been a beneficiary of the will, should not act as witnesses to the signing of a will. The doctor may have to be involved in certifying that the patient is of sound mind while signing any legal document. In any such situation the doctor must be satisfied that the patient understands the implications of what he is doing, at the time at which he is doing it, even if his understanding is shortlived as in the case of someone who is suffering from intermittent confusion.

Funeral arrangements

There may be many funeral directors, undertakers and staff at crematoria who are unwilling, through fear or ignorance, to deal with people with AIDS. The potential for distress to the partner, relatives or friends of patients will be reduced if the services of undertakers who have thought through the issues surrounding funeral arrangements for people with AIDS are used. Funeral directors may be able to advise as to which crematoria staff will deal sympathetically with the families and friends of those dying with AIDS. The families will often be extremely grateful and relieved to be able to take the advice of carers who have already set up good links with undertakers.

> A young man died at home having been cared for effectively by the primary care team. The district nurse suggested a well known local firm of undertakers to the family who were then left to contact the undertaker. When the men came to remove the body and found out that the patient had died from AIDS, they refused point-blank to take the body.

Such distressing situations may be avoided by carers exploring which of the local undertakers are willing to deal with people with AIDS. Families of people with AIDS may be relieved to be able to take the advice of carers who have established good arrangements with particular undertakers.

The National Association of Funeral Directors has dealt with the issues surrounding AIDS and do have well thought out policies. However, not all funeral directors accept or follow these.

People who have been receiving income support, unemployment benefit or housing benefits are entitled to assistance with funeral fees. The social worker or welfare assistant should be able to advise and help with arranging for this assistance. For patients who have died without funds of any sort it is possible to arrange a funeral through the local authority. Each local authority will have a contract with a particular undertaker and will use a specific crematorium so that there will be little choice. If a burial is wanted this may take place in a public grave which may hold up to eight adults. The funeral will take place at the discretion of the undertaker and will often, therefore, be in the early morning.

The transport of ashes or a body to another country may pose problems. Ashes being taken out in an urn will usually cause few problems and the undertaker will be able to advise. The funeral director or crematorium will have to supply a certificate of packaging and the death certificate should also be available. There may be different requirements for each country and a small fee may be payable. A container may be sent through the post, in which case a form of declaration has to be obtained from the crematorium and a customs declaration filled in. Again the funeral director will be able to advise.

Transporting a body from one country to another is likely to cause more problems, and the details should be explored and understood as far as possible before such a situation actually arises. It is important to know, for example, that if the body of a Jewish person is to be flown to Israel this has to be arranged so that the body arrives in time for burial within 24 hours of death. Jewish undertakers will know the details and links should have been set up with a local firm. Problems are most likely to arise at a weekend and it is important to have some emergency numbers available. Each country will have its own requirements and the appropriate consulate or embassy will be able to give the details of what is required for their country. Two certificates are generally required, one to be issued by the doctor involved in the care of the patient which declares that the body is not infectious, and a second certificate issued by the District Medical Officer to certify that there are no significant infectious diseases in the district. Most countries also have strict specifications for the coffin which has to be zinc lined; the rules are not so stringent if the body is going to Ireland and a few other countries such as Nigeria. Italy has particularly stringent specifications and this increases the overall cost of transporting a body to another country.

Viewing a body

When planning for terminal care in any hospital, hospice or sheltered accommodation it is important to plan for the viewing of a body after death, either in the patient's own room or in a separate room or small chapel of rest. Wherever viewing takes place it should be in quiet, dignified, and comfortable surroundings but where the body can be kept relatively cool for as long as possible. The body may be kept, with safety, in a cool environment for up to 12 hours (occasionally longer), enabling relatives and friends who have a distance to come to attend without undue pressure.

Body bags

In the United Kingdom guidelines specify that the body of someone who has died with AIDS should be placed in a body bag after death and not re-opened again. There does not appear to be any particular ogical or scientific reason for this, and in many other countries there are no such rules. Nurses who encounter this for the first time may find it extremely distressing to have to do and, of course, it can be very distressing for relatives and friends of the patient whose body has to be placed in the body bag. The bags themselves are made from semi-opaque heavy duty plastic in various sizes with a zip, and may be obtained from commercial firms; it is important to know who is the local supplier.

It is also important to have thought through the policy of the multi-professional team relating to the use of body bags. The body can be laid out as for any patient who has died, with viewing taking place before the body is wrapped in a sheet, placed into a body bag and removed by the undertakers. However, adherence to the DHSS guidelines can cause difficulties in fulfilling other legal requirements. If the body is to be cremated it has to be seen by two independent doctors. The first doctor is the patient's usual medical practitioner or the doctor who has cared for him during his terminal illness; the second doctor should be independent, i.e. not working in the same practice or team; he or she has, by law, to examine the body before filling in the second half of the cremation form. This means that the doctor has to unzip the body bag and unwrap at least part of the sheet in order to be able to fulfil the law as it is not usually possible for the second doctor to be available immediately after death; the second examination may take place a day or two later at the undertakers. It is really only necessary to use body bags when there is leakage of body fluids.

Accommodation for partners, family and friends

There are, as yet, very few hospices which will take people with AIDS; this may mean that those who do will of necessity have to take patients from a very wide catchment area. Hence, when planning for any institutional care of patients who are dying with AIDS, it is important to remember that many may have families who live a long way away, and that the families may have difficulty in finding accommodation at short notice. If possible, provision should be made to enable visitors to stay in or near the hospital, hospice, or wherever care is taking place. In planning accommodation it is also important to plan for support for the families or visitors who will be staying in that accommodation. It is extremely exhausting and draining for nurses who are caring for the patients to also be constantly supporting the relatives and friends of the dying patient. If no arrangements are made to enable relatives and friends to leave the ward or the unit and to find support through other team members, the full burden of their support falls onto the nursing staff, or sometimes even onto other patients and their visitors. This is, of course, not so in the home setting in the community. In this setting it may be helpful to make arrangements for relatives to meet with a counsellor, or with the doctor, or social worker in the health centre or in an office away from the home. It may be necessary to arrange for a volunteer or another member of the team to stay with the patient in order to give the family and carers a break, so that they themselves can go and find some relief or support outside the home and away from the patient.

When the patient is dying

In the final few days or weeks of a patient's life, it should be borne in mind by all, and at all times, that the overall aim of care is to enable the patient to die in comfort and dignity. There should be a continuing respect for the patient's wishes, even if he is unconscious. There should also be a respect for any religious requirements or needs that may have been expressed or which are implicit in the religion to which the patient belongs, for example, any last rites that are important to a Catholic, to a Jew or to a Muslim, or to a member of any other religious community. The person who has been caring for the patient could easily feel pushed out at this point by professionals who come in and take over, or by family members who may not, until then, have been much in evidence. The primary carer, if he or she should wish to be involved, should continue to give whatever care he or she feels able to give, cooperating with the nurse who may need to negotiate with the primary carer as to who does what. In hospitals care is usually given by the nurses; in hospices and in the home setting the families or partners are more frequently involved in the actual care of the patient. It may be necessary for the nurse to perform certain procedures, and it may be better for the carer and for the patient if the direct carer is not too closely involved particularly in some of the more distressing procedures, for example the dressing of a pressure sore or the giving of an enema.

As death approaches meticulous attention to detail is essential and communication between nurses and doctors in the monitoring of symptoms and responses to medication is of even greater importance than usual. It is important to plan for the provision of support and care for the family, partner, and friends as they grieve in anticipation and as they watch at the bedside. Plans should also be made to ensure that, if at all possible, the patient is not left alone at any time. A chaplain, priest or other religious leader, as appropriate, should be available both to the patient and to the family throughout, but a nurse or any other person may say a simple prayer of committal should this be wanted.

When the patient has died

Death must be ascertained and certified by a doctor, but when death is expected there is no need to await the doctor's arrival before laying out the body. However, before beginning any such procedure it is important to ensure that the wishes of the family are known. Cultural and religious practises must be respected and provision should be made for those who require a place in which to mourn or sit with the body for a prescribed length of time, such as 24 or 48 hours as is required in some religions. Such a place should be relatively private and perhaps even sound proof as there may be chanting or wailing taking place which may disturb other patients.

If the family are happy to allow the nurses to wash and dress the patient and to lay him out, this should be done in the family's choice of clothes. It should, of course, be done taking full body fluid precautions as there may be some leakage of body fluids. Any person who lays out the body should be issued with gloves and aprons. For the purpose of viewing, the body should be made to look comfortable, with the arms outside the sheet. The body should be placed in the body bag after all the viewing has taken place. As mentioned in the previous section 'In preparation', policies regarding these matters should have been thought through and the details decided upon before the nurse and mourners are faced with this situation.

The mourners may wish to be alone with the body for a while although the nurse or other professional involved should offer to stay with them should they wish it. They may wish also to discuss suitable local undertakers although, as already suggested, this matter may be better discussed when preparing for the imminent death. The health care professional who has been involved should liaise with the undertaker on behalf of the family, and should also arrange with the family when they wish to collect the death certificate which will be issued by the doctor. This may be on the following day and the next of kin or another representative of the family should take the death certificate to the Registrar of Births and Deaths to register the death as soon as possible.

The doctor should take care as to the wording on the death certificate (see also p. 45). It is likely to be extremely distressing for many families to see the word 'AIDS' spelt out. Where possible the wording on the certificate should be discussed with the family beforehand. Death certificates are not confidential documents, and are available for inspection by insurance companies etc. For correct statistical analysis and for planning purposes it is, of course, important that the cause of death is correctly reported, but the word AIDS should be avoided until health care professionals and society in general have stopped responding to the person with AIDS, or those who are linked to him, with fear, stigmatisation and discrimination.

It is important that those close to the person who has died are assured of continuing support and availability of the members of the caring team. The chaplain or minister of religion should be available for pastoral care and for discussion about funeral arrangements. The doctor should be available to the family, who may have questions or worries that they wish to discuss and there may be other practical matters to be dealt with. The interval between death and the funeral will be a fairly busy time with practical issues taking precedence over feelings. Bereavement support and follow up is very important at a later date and all those who are grieving should be reassured that this will be available to them when they need it. The health care professional should be aware that the bereaved person may need to express grief in tears, and should allow time and space for them to do so. Their need to express anger should also be accepted, remembering that the anger and sense of helplessness about the illness may well be displaced on to those who have been caring for the bereaved person's loved one. This anger should not be taken personally, although genuine cause for complaint should be investigated and dealt with. The whole team should be aware of and supportive of others throughout this time; one person should never be left alone to have to deal with several different groups of grieving people.

The good memories that people take away with them from this situation will depend, to a great extent, on the sensitivity with which the nurse and the doctor and any other members of the team deal with the small matters and details. For some it may be a simple prayer of committal that is said by the nurse at the time of death which will stand out in their memory and bring comfort. For others it will be the memory of a peaceful face, of being able to hold his hand and having that physical contact for the last time. For others it will be the inclusion of a poem or a special item such as a teddy bear or a 'Walkman' in the body bag before the body is taken away.

Some months after his partner's death, one man commented: 'The care that the team gave was very professional. They thought of everything. But what mattered most was the feeling of family which they created, the way in which we all shared in the caring and in the grieving.'

10 Intravenous drug use, AIDS and terminal care

In the UK there are still only a small number of intravenous drug users who have died with a diagnosis of AIDS. In Edinburgh where Dr Ray Brettle and his colleagues at the City Hospital have had a number of years of experience with drug users who are HIV positive, very few, as yet, have required terminal care. However, as those who are now HIV positive develop AIDS it is envisaged that many will need terminal care. In Edinburgh the majority of those who are now HIV positive or who are developing AIDS are in their late teens or early twenties, and a number are single parents with children who may or may not be HIV positive or have AIDS. The mothers and their children are being followed up by Dr J Mok who, together with Dr Brettle and other colleagues, run a family clinic enabling parents and children to be followed up together. The families of these young people will often look after them when they are ill at home, and some grand-parents are being left to look after small children.

Lothian region social services have been responsive and imaginative in planning for the continuing care of both adults and children with AIDS, or of children whose mothers are ill and in hospital or dying. Foster parents, adoptive parents, and landlords have been recruited and educated so that there are now a number of choices available to people with AIDS. For example, a prospective foster mother may be introduced to a mother who is likely to need repeated hospitalisation, so that a relationship is built up before the child needs to be fostered. This foster mother is then available on a 24 hour basis at any time should the mother need hospitalisation. This enables the mother to go into hospital knowing that her child will be taken care of by someone whom she trusts and knows. Some hospitals, including the City Hospital, have been flexible in allowing a mother and child to be admitted together, perhaps to the same ward or to different wards within the same hospital. However, when a mother is seriously ill she may not want or be able to cope with looking after an ill child. Some do not want their children to remember them looking very ill or dying.

Where drug addiction is endemic within a community, such as some housing estates, several members of the same family may be both intravenous drug users and be HIV positive. This, of course, puts a tremendous strain on the family, and members of that family may not be able to rely on each other to look after small children or someone who is terminally ill.

In any drug-using population the death rate is estimated to be 1 per cent per year. Some of these deaths will be accidental, some due to suicide, and some due to illness. It seems that there may be a small increase in the number of suicides in those who are HIV positive and drug using but, at present, the numbers are not thought to be significant. Dr Brettle, in a personal communication, described two patterns of response to the news that a drug user is HIV positive or has AIDS. Some become aggressively self-destructive and deteriorate dramatically; others suddenly find the motivation to improve their life-style and stop their drug use. John Atkinson, working in a community team with people with AIDS in Glasgow, suggests that there is a definite increase in self-destructive behaviour.

Clinically, drug users with AIDS present with recurrent or chronic chest problems, in particular bacterial pneumonias. Bacterial skin infections and other infections are extremely common. Most have had Hepatitis B, some will have chronic cirrhosis as a result, and in those with AIDS the Hepatitis B may be re-activated. Ten per cent of those who have Hepatitis B will, in any case, become carriers. Hepatitis D and Hepatitis C may also be current, and in those who have developed obvious signs of hepatitis but who are Hepatitis B negative, these may be the causative organism. All who are involved in the care of such patients should be vaccinated against Hepatitis B, and appropriate infection control measures should be taken.

There is also a 400 per cent increase in *Mycobacterium tuberculosis* causing pulmonary TB in drug users who are HIV positive. In the UK this is not resistant unless treatment has been inadequate and anti-tuberculous medication should continue as long as possible, or until death. Other patients should, of course, be protected from the person who is coughing and who has open TB, and staff should be Mantoux tested and, if necessary, vaccinated or followed up.

As with other people with AIDS, it is extremely difficult to define the terminal phase of the illness. Many will appear to be seriously ill or even moribund but will recover from that particular episode of infection. There may be a certain amount of negotiation or bargaining necessary when giving drugs related to pain control. Drug users may require higher doses than average to achieve the same result. However, in our experience there has been little difficulty in the patient who is seriously or terminally ill. The problems arise when the patient recovers. As the patient becomes weaker and closer to death the problems related to their drug addiction appear to become irrelevant. The patient's pain should be treated as necessary – if it is adequately treated there will be few problems. The normal principles of prophylactic pain control and titration of dosages should be followed in the terminal care situation.

Acknowledgements

Dr R Brettle and Dr J Mok, City Hospital, Edinburgh, Scotland; Dr D Wollner, Beth Abram Hospice Programme, New York, USA; and Dr J Strang, Maudsley Hospital DDU, London, UK.

11 Terminal care for women and children with AIDS

> Karen is three years old. She has come into hospital for her three-weekly infusion of gamma globulin. In the cot next to her is two year old Emma. They and their parents know each other well as they have been coming in like this every three weeks since each was nine months old.
>
> Karen and Emma are both quite small for their age with big hollow eyes, thin hair and dry skin. Karen accepts the hospital routine quite passively including the infusion needle in her arm. The infusion over, Karen is enjoying a bowl of strawberry ice cream whilst the paediatrician is talking to her mother. The doctor is explaining that she is going to give Karen Zidovudine. Her 'T' helper cell count is very low and the doctor is worried that Karen's immune system is going to be overcome and that she will then deteriorate very quickly. Karen's mother wonders whether she should be having Zidovudine as well; she also has AIDS. She is feeling very tired and is very worried about what will happen to Karen if she is ill and cannot look after her, or if she dies before Karen does.

Children with AIDS

In the United Kingdom the number of children who have AIDS is still relatively small. Most of these children will be cared for, and ultimately die, in hospital. A few may die at home cared for by their parent(s) with back-up from the Primary Care team and/or specialist home care teams.

The modes of transmission in children are
— from a mother who is HIV antibody positive; and
— through receiving contaminated blood and blood products.

Children with AIDS commonly suffer from the following.
— *Pneumocystis carinii* pneumonia or lymphoid interstitial pneumonitis which cause dyspnoea and pyrexia.
— Candidiasis which may be recurrent and severe and cause difficulty with eating, as may herpes sores in and around the mouth.
— Intractable diarrhoea and severe weight loss.
— Recurrent opportunistic and bacterial infections.
— CNS involvement and encephalopathy may be evident in retarded

development, spasticity, weakness and fits. (These children often
need long term care.)
— Failure to thrive.

Input to care for these children will be as for any child with a life
threatening illness – an appropriate response to the individual needs of
the child and his or her family. It is essential that the carers have a
knowledge and understanding of paediatric AIDS, symptom control
and palliative care. As many of the babies and children will have a
mother with HIV disease, issues relating to fostering and adoption must
be explored and options identified.

At the present time it is both possible and appropriate for children
with AIDS to be cared for either in hospital or at home. There are,
however, several factors that need to be considered if health care professionals are to continue to be able to respond effectively to the needs
of these children and their families, as numbers grow.

— The long term needs of children who are chronically sick.
— The fact that many mothers do not want to care for their children
  'at home'. 'Home' may be a squat or bed and breakfast accommodation.
— Some mothers will be 'chaotic' drug users and be unable to care
  for a sick child.
— Chronically ill mothers with well or sick children will need help
  and respite.

The experience of colleagues in New York caring for large numbers of
children with AIDS, indicate that it is necessary to plan to provide long
term care for children. Terminal care facilities for children, as a back
up to community care, may also be needed. Planners of services within
the statutory and voluntary sector need to talk to mothers who are HIV
antibody positive, and carers already involved, to try to identify what
will be required and any likely gaps in service provision.

Women with AIDS

Women may acquire the human immunodeficiency virus through:
— sharing needles and syringes with an infected person
— having sexual intercourse with an infected person
— receiving infected blood or blood products
— following organ transplants or insemination by infected donor
  semen.
As with children, the number of women with AIDS who have died in
this country is still relatively small. The clinical management of adults
is very similar whether they are male or female, bearing in mind that
care must be individually tailored to needs. However, a particular need

for women is for facilities that allow children to stay with their mother, and for families to stay together when they need to. Within the remit of continuing care there is a need for

— respite care for mothers – if they have children they may decide to leave them with a friend or family member if they have one, or bring them with them;

— rehabilitative care following acute illness (with or without children);

— terminal care for women (with or without children);

— respite care for chronically ill children (with or without mother).

At a discussion with a group of women who were HIV antibody positive, the group said they know of over 300 women in the London area who were HIV antibody positive and many of them had been ill. The following comments were made:

'If you think we want to be cared for at home, you're wrong. Home is prison for lots of us'.

'Can we have a day at the day centre for women only?'

'I don't want to be with men; men are bad news when you're ill, they clear off.'

'I don't want my little one to see me when I'm dying, would that be O.K.?'

'Try to look after a screaming toddler when you're feeling this tired, it's hell.'

'We need somewhere where we can have a break every now and then. Then we can carry on.'

'Sometimes I'm so scared, but I don't tell anyone; you can't can you?'

Efforts to keep children with their ill mothers are now successfully made in several hospitals, and the need for families to stay together is clearly recognised, as is the need to address issues such as adoption and fostering and the long term care of children with AIDS. The operation of a 'fixed foster parent scheme' (see p. 97) may remove some of the anxieties women feel about their child being fostered by strangers.

Julie's story

Julie was in the day room of a hospital, sitting on the edge of a chair smoking a cigarette. She was asked by the doctor if she would return to her room so that we could talk with her about her referral to Mildmay. Julie, a young girl of 25 attempted to walk – she was stooped, wasted and so weak that the doctor had to almost carry her. When she got to her bed it took some time as she climbed on to the bed determined to do it on her own – her 'non-verbals' made this very clear. Once there she listened whilst the doctor told her about Mildmay, all the while eyeing me with the greatest suspicion.

'Will I have my own room?' 'What's the food like?'
'Can I smoke?' 'Are the people there friendly?'
'Will I get my methadone?'

As she sat there, her large blue eyes staring from such a small face she reminded me of a waif, a stray, so vulnerable, so insecure.

Julie's background

Julie was the second of five children. She had three brothers, who all attended schools for educationally sub-normal children, and one sister. Julie was the most intelligent member of the family and found that position difficult. She did not make any effort at school as it would only widen the gap between her and her family.

Julie was seven years old when her sister was born, and soon afterwards her mother had a nervous breakdown. Over the next two years Julie's mother took five overdoses and slashed her wrists.

When Julie was 11 years old she was brought before the Juvenile Court for non-attendance at school – she had been staying at home to protect her younger sister. By the age of 13 she had run away from home four times and belonged to a group of 'greasers'. Julie admitted to having sexual intercourse with over a dozen men, some of whom she refused to name. There were strong suspicions that members of her family were involved and that was thought to be the reason why she felt the need to protect her sister.

At 12 years of age Julie was encouraged, by her parents, to dye her hair, paint her finger and toe nails, wear heavy make-up and was also permitted to smoke. She once said she would rather have been a boy – they have more choices – she seldom wore dresses, mostly jeans and dungarees.

Julie was in institutional care for most of her early teens. She had her first pregnancy terminated and was given the pill when she was 13 years of age. It was recorded that Julie had often been involved in fights and had often been 'kicked in'.

At the age of 16 Julie came to London and became addicted to heroin. She funded this by prostitution and theft. At the age of 17 she gave birth to a son who was immediately adopted. She had one particular boy friend 'on and off' over the following years and also became involved in what was, to her, a very meaningful same sex relationship. She lived in squats and said that her friends disappeared when she first became ill.

Julie's illness

In 1987, for several months Julie was in and out of London hospitals suffering from weakness, malaise, and inability to cope with her numerous social problems. In June of 1987 she was diagnosed as HIV antibody positive although admitted initially with a diagnosis of pelvic inflammatory disease.

In January 1988 she had PCP (*Pneumocystis carinii* pneumonia) and

began to deteriorate generally. She developed episodes of Meningo
Encephalitis. It was concluded that this was the direct effect of the HIV
infection.

Julie in Mildmay

On admission to Mildmay Julie was very quiet, withdrawn and passive.
She was very thin, having lost a lot of weight. Her hair was sparse, and
had recently been infested with head lice. Her skin was dry and coarse.
She was occasionally incontinent of urine, and was weak and unsteady
on her feet. She had oral and oesophageal candida and was on oral
Ketocanazole, nystatin and Acyclovir.

She had last used Heroin nine months before and was now on Methadone (3 mgs bd). She asked if she had AIDS. She said she did not know
she had AIDS and quickly changed the subject. Was this denial? Was
this short-term memory loss?

When she was asked about family and friends she said she did not
wish to talk about them and anyway they would not want to know her
now she had AIDS.

She had her own supply of vodka and smoked 20–30 cigarettes a day.
Initially she kept asking for diamorphine, and then for increases in her
Methadone. She complained of not feeling very well and attributed
everything to not having enough Methadone. When she had settled in
her need for Methadone was variable. After one month she decided she
would wean herself off the Methadone and although doses were always
offered she refused everything except for very few occasions.

Julie settled quite quickly but was very suspicious at first. She seemed
to prefer to talk to the older women on the staff, perhaps they represented
the mother figure she had never had. She was very frightened. Frightened
of
— being alone
— rejection
— dying alone which led to her being frightened of falling asleep alone
— she was afraid of going to hell.
Her fear of rejection showed itself in the way that she would never ask
anyone to sit with her; rather, as you walked in, she would say 'Don't
you want a bloody chair then?'

Julie would go in and out of denial about her condition, coping as
best she could on different occasions! As she got to know and trust
people, she loved being held and cuddled and would often only sleep if
her hand was held and a promise was made not to leave her. Julie needed
someone to be there, not to do or listen, but just a presence. Her wishes
were respected and even when unconscious she was not left on her
own.

Julie would often tell staff she was afraid of death, not dying but death.
She talked with several members of the team including the chaplain,
counsellor, doctors and several nurses about her fears. Her main fear was
that she might go to hell. She said she would like to know about 'religion',
was it too late for her? She was reassured of God's love for her. She
asked people to pray with her and for her, but she could not bear 'Our
Father'. She asked, 'What will it be like when I die?' On being told that

we believed she would be with God, which would be better than anything she had ever known, she became much calmer. She often asked for the 23rd Psalm to be read to her and this seemed to soothe her fears.

In an atmosphere of love and security Julie was free to share her fears and pain, but it was in her time and at her initiation. She talked with the counsellor about her funeral service and chose Psalm 23 and her favourite hymns; and during this time she put many of her personal affairs in order.

Two months after her admission her general condition started to deteriorate quite rapidly. She had been becoming weaker for days, had become incontinent, complaining of severe pains. She was diagnosed as having a chronic aseptic meningitis, probably due to HIV.

It became necessary to give her oral morphine as she entered the terminal phase of her illness. Later she was started on diamorphine via a syringe driver and Nozinan and Hyocine were added.

Ten weeks after Julie was admitted to Mildmay she died. She had been deeply unconscious for several days.

Mildmay had become her home and the staff her family. Apart from her sister and her one good friend she had no-one else. It seemed appropriate, and the wish of Julie and her friend, that the funeral go from Mildmay and the mourners return there. Julie's mother and brother came to the funeral invited by the sister.

It was a privilege to care for Julie and we are grateful to her for all she taught us about attitudes and caring, and for the glimpse she gave us into the experience, environment and world of one woman with AIDS.

Acknowledgements

Dr Diana Gibb and Ms Candy Duggan at The Hospital for Sick Children, Great Ormond Street, London; Dr Jacqueline Mok and Dr Ray Brettle, The City Hospital, Edinburgh; Body Positive (Women's Group); and Positively Women.

12   Conclusion

As we look at the terminal care needs of people with AIDS and at the ways in which we might appropriately respond to them, we are reminded again of the real people who taught us most of what we know. Robert, Julie, Mark, Andrew, Martin and many more, allowed us to share with them at a very special time in their lives, and in so doing challenged our attitudes, assumptions, and ways of caring. In the changing and developing climate of care for people with AIDS, we still have so much to learn. It is an on-going process. As the epidemic spreads in the heterosexual community, and more women and children are affected, we must continue to address issues relating to their special needs. We must be pro-active, planning for our provision, not waiting until we have to react, often inadequately, to crisis situations.

Further reading

References cited within the text are given at the end of the particular chapter.

Clinical and nursing

AIDS

Adler, M. W. (Ed.) (1987). *ABC of AIDS*. British Medical Journal, London.

Farthing, C. (1986). *A Colour Atlas of AIDS*. Wolfe Publishing Ltd, London.

Farthing, C. Brown, S. and Staughton, R. (1988). *A Colour Atlas of AIDS and HIV Disease*, second edition. Wolfe Publishing Ltd, London.

Friedman-Kein, A. E. (1988). *Colour Atlas of AIDS*. W. B. Saunders, London.

Miller, D., Webber, J. and Cress, J. (1986). *The Management of AIDS patients*. Macmillan, Basingstoke.

Pratt, R. (1991). *AIDS: A Strategy for Nursing Care*, third edition. Edward Arnold, London.

Rosenblum, M. L., Levy, R. M. and Bredesen, D. E. (1988). *AIDS and the nervous system*. Raven Press, New York.

Royal College of Nursing (1986). *Nursing Guidelines on the Management of Patients in Hospital and the Community suffering from AIDS*. Scutari Press, London.

Youle, M., Farthing, C., Clarbour, J. and Wade, P. (1988). *AIDS: Therapeutics in HIV Disease*. Churchill Livingstone, Edinburgh.

General

Bates, T. D., Duncan, W., Ellis, H., Sikora, K. *et al* (Eds). *Clinical Oncology. Contemporary Palliation of Difficult Symptoms*. Balliere, London.

Manning, M. (1984). *The Hospice Alternative. Living with Dying*. Souvenir Press, London.

Munley, A. (1983). *The Hospice Alternative. A new context for death and dying*. Basic Books, London.

Swerdlow, M. and Ventafridda, V. (Eds). (1987). *Cancer Pain*. MTP Press Ltd, Lancaster, UK.
Twycross, R. and Lack, S. (1990). *Therapeutics in Terminal Cancer*, second edition. Churchill Livingstone, Edinburgh.

Social, Counselling and Pastoral

AIDS

Green, J. (1989). *Counselling in HIV infection and AIDS*. Blackwell Scientific Publications, Oxford.
Kirkpatrick, B. (1988). *AIDS: Sharing the Pain*. Darton, Longman and Todd, London.
Kubler-Ross, E. (1987). *AIDS: The Ultimate Challenge*. Macmillan, Basingstoke.
Miller, D. (1987). *Living with AIDS and HIV*. Macmillan, Basingstoke.
Miller, R. and Bor, R. (1988). *AIDS: A guide to clinical counselling*. Science Press, London.
Oyler, C. and Oyler, J. (1988). *Go Toward the Light*. Harper and Rowe, London.
Shilts, R. (1988). *And the band played on*. Penguin Books, Harmondsworth, Middlesex.

General

Ainsworth-Smith, I. and Speck, P. (1982). *Letting Go*. Society for the Promotion of Christian Knowledge, London.
Cassidy, S. (1988). *Sharing the Darkness*. Darton, Longman and Todd, London.
Foskett, J. and Lyall, D. (1988). *Helping the helpers – supervision and pastoral care*. Society for the Promotion of Christian Knowledge, London.
Government White Paper. (1989). *Caring for People – Community care in the next decade and beyond*. CM849. HMSO, London.
Kubler-Ross, E. (1982). Living with death and dying. Souvenir Press, London.
McGilloway, O. and Myco, F. (1985). *Nursing and Spiritual Care*. Harper and Row, London.
Neuberger, J. (1987). *Caring for Dying People of different faiths*. Austen Cornish, London.
Speck, R. (1988). *Being there – pastoral care in time of illness*. Society for the Promotion of Christian Knowledge, London.

Women's issues

Richardson, D. (1989). *Women and the AIDS Crisis*, second edition. Pandora Press, London.

Drug Misuse/Abuse and AIDS

Advisory Council on the Misuse of Drugs (1984). *Report*. HMSO, London.

Advisory Council on the Misuse of Drugs (1988). *AIDS and Drug Misuse*. HMSO, London.

Banks, A. and Waller, T. A. M. (1988). *Drug Misuse – A Practical Handbook for General Practitioners*. Blackwell Scientific Publications, Oxford.

Brettle, R. P. (1987). *Evidence to the Working Party on AIDS and Drug Misuse*. Advisory Council on Misuse of Drugs. HMSO, London.

Brettle, R. P., Bisset, K., Burns, S. *et al.* (1987). Human immunodeficiency virus and drug abuse: the Edinburgh experience. *British Medical Journal*, **295**, 421–4.

Bulkin, W., Brown, L., Fraioli, D. (1988). Hospice care for the intravenous drug user – AIDS patients in a skilled nurse facility. *Journal of Acquired Immuno-deficiency*, **1**, 375–80.

Roberton, J. R., Bucknill, A. B. V, Wellsby, P. D. *et al.* (1986). An epidemic of AIDS related virus (HTLV–III/LAV) injection amongst intravenous drug abusers in Scottish general practice. *British Medical Journal*, **292**, 527–30.

Robertson, A. R. (1987). *Heroin, AIDS and Society*. Hodder and Stoughton, Sevenoaks, Kent.

Appendix 1

Useful addresses (correct in August 1990).

AIDS Care Education and Training (ACET)
PO Box 1323
London   W5 5TF
Telephone (081) 840 7879

Body Positive
PO Box 493
London   W14 0TF
Telephone (071) 835 1045

British Humanist Association
14 Lamb's Conduit Passage
London   WC1R 4RH
Telephone (071) 430 0908

The British Red Cross
Beautycare and Cosmetic Camouflage Department
National Headquarters
9 Grosvenor Crescent
London   SW1X 7EJ
Telephone (071) 235 5454
(Beautycare organisers are available at local county branches.)

Cruse
Cruse House
126 Sheen Road
Richmond
Surrey   TW9 1UR
Telephone (081) 940 4818

Frontliners
55 Farringdon Road
London   EC1M 3JB
Telephone (071) 430 1199

The London Lighthouse
111–117 Lancaster Road
London   W11 1QT
Telephone (071) 792 1200

Mainliners
PO Box 125
London   SW9 8EF
Telephone (071) 274 4000 Ext. 354

Mildmay Mission Hospital
Hackney Road
London   E2 7NA
Telephone (071) 739 2331

Positive Partners
10 Rathbone Place
London W1
Telephone (071) 249 6068

Positively Women
333 Grays Inn Road
London WC1X 8PX
Telephone (071) 837 9705

The Terrence Higgins Trust (THT)
52–54 Grays Inn Road
London   WC1X 8JU
Telephone (071) 831 0330; Helpline (071) 242 1010

Appendix 2

Check list of benefits available for people with AIDS/HIV

Employed or Self-employed
Fit for Work

Family Credit
Housing Benefit
Mobility Allowance
Attendance Allowance
Social Fund – Crisis Loans

Employed or Self-employed *Unfit for Work*	Statutory Sick Pay (SSP) Sickness Benefits Invalidity Benefit (after 28 weeks) Income Support Housing Benefit Mobility Allowance Attendance Allowance Social Fund Payments
Not Employed (Have sufficient National Insurance Contributions) *Fit for Work*	Unemployment Benefit Income Support Housing Benefit Mobility Allowance Attendance Allowance Social Fund Payments
Not Employed (Have sufficient National Insurance Contributions) *Unfit for Work*	Sickness Benefit Invalidity Benefit (after 28 weeks) Income Support Housing Benefit Mobility Allowance Attendance Allowance Social Fund Payments
Not Employed (Insufficient Contributions paid) e.g. people who have not worked for sometime	Income Support Housing Benefits Mobility Allowance Attendance Allowance Social Fund Payments
Not Employed (Insufficient Contributions paid) *Unfit for Work*	Income Support Severe Disablement Allowance (after 28 weeks) Housing Benefits Mobility Allowance Attendance Allowance Social Fund Payments

Index